Trapped
in Silence

Dedication

From the depth of my heart and very being this book is my
gift to the pure wonder that is my brother Daniel, who does
not know the meaning of jealousy.

I LOVE YOU WITH EVERYTHING THAT I AM, ALWAYS

Written especially from the endless love that I have for my
precious family and many treasured friends whose faith and
encouragement made many things possible.

I WOULD BE NOTHING WITHOUT YOU AND MY LIFE WOULD BE SO
EMPTY, TOO

Portrayed with eternal thoughts of gratitude to the splendour
of all Australians who lifted my soul simply because they took
the time to care.

WE ARE THE LUCKY COUNTRY

Inspired by the courageous spirit of fellow disabled people
and their loved ones of the past and present who pave an
easing path for me to follow.

TOGETHER WE WILL TEACH LOVE AND UNDERSTANDING

Trapped in Silence

The autobiography of a remarkable young man

BRADLEY HARRIS WOLF

BANTAM BOOKS
SYDNEY • AUCKLAND • TORONTO • NEW YORK • LONDON

TRAPPED IN SILENCE

A BANTAM BOOK

First published in Australia and New Zealand in 1994 by Bantam

National Library of Australia.
Cataloguing-in-Publication Entry.

Wolf, Bradley Harris, 1977–.
  Trapped in silence.

  ISBN 1 86359 260 1.

  1. Wolf, Bradley Harris, 1977–. 2. Cerebral palsied —
Australia — Biography. 3. Cerebral palsied — Australia —
Means of communication. I. Title.

362.1968360092

Bantam Books are published by

Transworld Publishers (Aust) Pty Limited
15-25 Helles Avenue, Moorebank, NSW 2170

Transworld Publishers (NZ) Limited
3 William Pickering Drive, Albany, Auckland

Transworld Publishers (UK) Limited
61-63 Uxbridge Road, Ealing, London W5 5SA

Bantam Doubleday Dell Publishing Group Inc
1540 Broadway, New York, New York 10036

Edited by Marie-Louise Taylor
Cover design by Reno Design Group 12500
Cover photograph by Murray Ware
Text design by Reno Design Group
Typeset by Bookset Pty Ltd
Printed by Australian Print Group
Production by Vantage Graphics, Sydney
10 9 8 7 6 5 4 3 2 1

Contents

To Ena Gibbs

Oh my darling grandmama

where do you find the stamina

to work for hours at the farm

yet cradle me in your loving arm

with so much love in your heart

after an early morning start

No matter how tired you may be

you always have a smile for me

there's love for me in your eyes

that's something you can't disguise

Don't ever change, my lovely one

for the love's returned by your grandson.

Foreword

Bradley Wolf is my friend. I admire, respect and love him. I first met Bradley a few years ago after he wrote to me. Pam Provost, a close friend of Bradley's and executive co-ordinator of the charity he founded, Silence Isn't Golden, rang and asked me if I would like to meet him when he and his Mum came to stay with her in Sydney. I knew a little about cerebral palsy, having met some other kids who suffered from it, and I was not going to be fazed by what his medical condition might present. I knew also that these 'special' people have a natural and giving way; affection seems to come easily to them.

Of course, I didn't know what to expect from Brad himself so I was naturally nervous. I knew from his letter that he was a gifted writer. As a writer myself I'm always impressed by anyone who can write in such a way that moves me emotionally. But Bradley is truly gifted not just as a writer, but in a total sense. He is in my opinion a total human being. He is acutely aware of his physical existence and all that this entails and at the same time he is in direct contact with his spiritual self. His twisted body houses a mind and spirit of a quality which few of us attain in one lifetime. I strive daily to be like Bradley. He is an inspiration. He gives me courage, he gives me his friendship and he gives me his love. Thank you, Brad.

Your friend always,

Angry Anderson

Acknowledgements

This book was published by a house who I admire and have great respect for as their reputation and belief in me is unforgettable. They instil much honour within this ordinary teenager who has been given the chance he always dreamed of.

Now that this opportunity has knocked I won't complain about the noise.

I offer my heartfelt thanks to those who stood by me and fought for my rights and my quality of life. They gave me everything by teaching me how to love when all I wanted to do was hate.

I appreciate you being there for me.

The glory is yours.

May those who put the fire in my heart by sending many beautiful cards and letters of congratulations when I began to communicate know that their messages of hope are my most cherished possessions. I extend my deepest admiration for your wonderful generosity in giving just for joy. I'm humbled by the children's patience in awaiting a reply to their tributes and feel truly blessed by their gentility and thoughtfulness in making allowances in regard to my time and ability. But most of all I thank them for not expecting perfection from me.

When I sometimes think I can't

all I have to do is remember your words

and know that any challenge is worth the effort.

Finally, I pray with sincerity that what I have to say makes a difference, if only to one, in our individual search to see our God smile upon us for being the best we can be at this very moment, thus loving us perfectly so much more than we love ourselves and those around us. I thank Him for the obstacles which have made me stronger and made me a better person, and for my disability for through that I have found my purpose. Everything that has happened was a part of His awesome plan.

We are not here to find God;

he is always there with open arms.

We are here to find ourselves.

Preface

Welcome to my solitary universe where life was once buried but blossomed with laughter in my prison of a rebellious body that stored my mind but never shielded the wisdom of forgiveness nor sheltered the feelings of my love for all mankind. My body is now free. Nothing is impossible if we believe in ourselves and miracles. Never give up on your dreams but give praise for everything for all is not lost with positive thinking. We create and form our own life with our thoughts and choices for what we need to know at a particular point in time. No-one else is to blame for we are all absolutely responsible for ourselves, and a thought is so easily changed — time is the essence.

None of us are perfect

but we can try to be

and if at first we don't succeed

we have to try again

No matter what you want, be happy.

I was never truly anybody until I loved someone and I do worship the very ground that my mum and dad walk on, side by side with my truest mate, Danny. I can always count on them. I became the one with all the glory but they were the ones with all the strength; their unwavering devotion is my inspiration and peace of mind for they led me away from bitterness, chaos and pain. To have their love and to give them mine is my reason for living.

There isn't anything I wouldn't do for my beloved grandparents. If it meant their happiness I'd gladly die for them but not before they knew that nobody can ever take their place where I keep them in my heart. My only wish is to tell them that their unconditional love is returned with everything that is their grandson.

My uncles Colin and Robert were always there for me and treated me like a son. They only wanted to give me the best; they did, for I had them. I don't cry as much as I did before as they removed the sadness and put laughter in my eyes and a smile upon my face. Now that they are older and have children of their own I haven't been forgotten for they still accept me as I am. And now I have two beautiful aunties to adore. Peta and Sylvia not only opened up their minds; they greeted me with their hearts. I've never felt anything so perfect as the affection my little cousins Rebecca, Ashleigh, Taylah and Blake, give. They are growing up in an ever-changing but more receptive society with wonderful parents who know that children are a reflection of their own behaviour so endeavour to make a precious life safe and secure. Yet they still have time to love me like they do.

Even though I do not share the same bloodlines as Nanny and Poppy Wolf, they have still touched me with their serenity. They recognise me and care for me as if I was their grandson. To them I am; they don't reject my love, in fact they send it back tenfold and are not concerned about anything except my felicity and health. My Poppy is not able to share my conquests but he also does not have to hide the pain of cancer any more as he is at peace now. We miss him every day yet know that he will never leave us for he lives in our hearts with the many glorious memories that only he could leave behind. Through my Poppy I learnt to honour my body, however it may be, and how to smile to shield the pain that I don't want to show.

I see so much of them in my Uncle Graeme. Although he is his own person, he shares their many relaxed and thought-provoking ways. When I was too sick to care and my parents' finances were swallowed up, he did not hesitate to send his savings and never worried about being repaid — money was the last thing on his mind as long as I grew well again. My other uncle, Gary, together with his wife Linda and their sons Toby and Benjamin, all have the knack that it takes to be a special friend. Whenever they are near, good times are not far behind.

Graeme and Gary's sister, Sylvia, has what it takes to make the world shine with her naive and passive ways for it takes little or nothing just to make her smile. I am not the only one who appreciates her finer attributes as my Uncle Colin has the pleasure of her being his wife. It is pure heaven entering their home as I feel the rush of love meeting me at the door. They've brought so much out of each other, I couldn't ask for more.

I will always be grateful to my natural father for giving me this life and thankful to my loved ones who taught me how to enjoy it. My father Ian has taken a separate path for almost all my years but that doesn't mean I love him any less and all I can hope is that he has found his happiness. My paternal grandparents and Uncle Neil and Aunt Wendy seemingly are not meant to be an instrumental part of my journey for I have only had intermittent contact with them, mostly before I can remember. But to me they are a vital part of my heritage which I enfold with the richest parts of me. I can only assume they care about me in their own way for who I am. I understand that they may have regrets about my situation. It meant a lot to me when Grandpa Pat, while on holidays, came to visit both Danny and me. My door will always be open to all the Harris family.

The rest of my large and loving family, whether they be a Clifford, Gibbs, Harris or Wolf, all showered me with many joyous moments which kept my silent hopes aflame and even now bring a glow to my heart when I think of them again. The miles may separate us but we're joined at the heart for God brought us together. This is my chance to communicate to these loved ones and let them know that they are forever on my mind, for how could I ever toss aside the Christmas spirit they carry with them the whole year through. To most of them it never mattered that some of their ways don't work for me, as we all know that most of mine aren't their cup of tea, but we did what we wanted and were who we needed to be and went on loving each other just the same.

Without the special brand of dedicated teachers, led by Anne and Kerry Dickson, who were trained to guide me well, none of what we did in the short time I spent in formal education would have been accomplished. Because they weren't afraid to overstep the mark and walk away from the comfort zone by taking a chance on me, we were able to succeed in what we'd set our minds to do. They were willing to take a million to one chance on me, and they didn't care that I wasn't a genius or want the surety of a child prodigy for they just respected the fact that I wanted to learn.

Their risks and commitment helped unchain the tag of a fool that many thought I wore. Confidence was one of the greatest gifts that the teachers and the students at my schools gave me. One of them, in particular, Rebecca Irvine, is still a very good friend to me.

For years I couldn't find the key to open up my silent world and just when I was about to give up hope, along came technology and many dreams just fell into place for I was to be one of the lucky ones who would be set free. On that memorable day in January 1991 I wrote my first message to the world: 'I love you, Dad'. After that nothing could stop me.

I've never known what was around the corner but I learnt so much sitting on the sidelines; I just had to be a good listener. I discovered many things, mainly about myself. I discovered how prejudiced and selfish I could be. We are all different, whether we are disabled or not. I share a similar affliction to many who simply have a twisted frame but even our distorted fingerprints separate us, as does our given name. Of course our degree of brain damage varies; some of my disabled friends are able to walk and talk while some go home to heaven without ever openly expressing themselves. But each and every one of them is here for a reason, to fulfil a purpose and give what only he or she can offer. We all have a right to live; it doesn't matter if we're black or white, able-bodied or disabled, our tears all look alike. Now that I can communicate I can only speak for myself and be entirely contented with all that I have.

Within two hours of writing my first message, after a clear request from my headmaster Kerry Dickson, the Queensland Alumina Sports Club sent around their president, Gary Frost, who stood at my door with a grin from ear to ear and a promise of a donated computer to use at home until my final year. They didn't expect Australia to hear about their goodwill but on that day in January 1991 they didn't just give me a keyboard with a screen attached, they gave my family a personality that many assumed was lost. The death sentence hovering overhead was substituted with a determination to grow stronger and say what was locked inside for so long, with many pent up dreams coming to the fore.

During the thirteen years of being trapped in silence very seldom did I receive personal mail. However, after the *Glad-stone Observer, Courier Mail* and Channel Ten so eloquently spread the news, hundreds of letters flooded in. Each unsealed envelope touched places inside me where faith had not been seen. I'll forever be indebted to all media networks as they portrayed my life with the utmost dignity and class. Although I felt my story wasn't out of the ordinary — every community is filled with stories — I was overwhelmed by the fact that no journalist sensationalised the truth. I have the highest regard for and value the courtesy and professionalism of Juanita Phillips, Walter Murray, Jim Brown, Katrina Lee, John Mangos, Werner Russell, Scott Jones, John Laws, Des McWilliam and our local reporter John Felix, along with the teams behind them, as they were instrumental in allowing many marvels to unfold. I wasn't just another story to them; they became my friends. As much as I desire to give credit where it's due by naming all the people who have helped me along the way, I know they will understand that it's not feasible and are enriched that their kindly deeds have touched many lives. I and many others will never forget what you have done.

The people who grew to know me after reading or hearing the news knew that I wanted to go to Disneyland and had sent a donation, wanting it to be more. The force of their generosity was overwhelming and I couldn't deny them the pleasure of giving. So their donations went towards the establishment of the Silence Isn't Golden foundation to create some practical wonders for the thousands of other Bradley stories out there. I know how expensive equipment can be and that most carers cannot afford it or don't have the luxury of donated devices to untwist or unearth someone special. Medication, therapy and the endless necessities devour a wage and, as welcome as a handicap allowance is, it is minimal compared to the costs. My scripts that alleviate the pain alone nearly eat a salary each month, but thanks to the NHS scheme the once almost impossible task of servicing my needs is diminished and I'm sure that many other imperative facilities are on the way. Unfortunately in these lean times even charitable organisations have for some time had to reduce the amount of help they can give. Carers or disabled people must now make up the difference. The charities do their best with what they've got during this decade where charity begins at home. Nowadays there are so many worthy organisations beating at the door, but whatever one tugs at your heartstrings please know that a little amounts to a lot. Fund raising isn't an easy chore but it is the most rewarding experience. I believe, however, that it's appalling that disabled people not only have to overcome a handicap but strive to purchase very expensive equipment.

I won't allow myself to focus on the downside, thus the Silence Isn't Golden foundation was born. My aim was to make another's life a little easier and, with the help of others, I used the funds sent to me to donate specialised devices so that not only my goals could be fulfilled. I don't want to promise miracles or give false hope to people who have been hurt enough, but so far in two and a half years, thirty-six people on an ever-growing waiting list have received computers or Unitems muscle stimulators. Of that small group three children are no longer as dependent on wheelchairs, two other children have communicated to their family, who were told that it couldn't be done, and all of them want to abundantly thank those responsible for giving them the answers to their prayers. There is a little boy who waited two years for a wheelchair; thanks to the goodwill of a lovely Darwin couple he is mobile again. So, as you can see, I got much more than what Disneyland has to offer as I found the place where I belong doing what I enjoy the most.

But it doesn't end there for the grandest aspect of all is that I met a beautiful friend named Pam. There isn't a thing in the world she wouldn't do for me and I treasure each magic moment when Pam Provost is with me. She is a part of my family and it is so wonderful to have a friend so rare and true whose support and hard work shine through. She doesn't want public acclaim but simply the opportunity to heal another's life. Pam devotes many hours to overseeing the Silence Isn't Golden foundation as a business without receiving a wage. Pam is the marketing manager for the Hancotronic Company which supplies Unitems electronic muscle stimulator machines. The company helps to cover the administration costs so that every tax deductible donation can go straight to those in need. Her enthusiasm alone makes me want to live and one day walk. Anyway, I don't imagine St Peter would allow two larrikins of our calibre to enter. I don't want to go as I'd miss her dancing eyes and all the other things we've laughed and cried over. This lovely lady with a colourful life makes each experience much lighter with her wit. During our fund-raising ventures we've at times done it tough and our dreams don't just happen, but simply being near her makes my spirits rise.

We would achieve very little without the tireless volunteers and ever-giving sponsors who bequeath their all to the Silence Isn't Golden foundation. We might be a land of battlers but I'm more than proud to be a part of it. Australia was shaped by characters of extraordinary insight who show that a down-under mate will always lend a helping hand.

Writing this book has been very therapeutic for me as I was nervous at the thought of releasing my pent up feelings and revealing how imperfect I can be. As my desires form into context I now know why I named a charity the way I did and when the day comes that I can halt my fault-finding ways to feel and say only nice things about another then I should remember that sometimes silence *is* golden. Those who know much say little but those who know little say much.

Pam's daughters are a credit to their upbringing and the moment we met they gave their unquestioning friendship and respect for who I am. Yet they know that they shine brightly in my heart, because I told them so. Yasmin and Melissa Oliveri are the sisters I never had. Even if I did I doubt that my feelings would be greater than what I have for those two beautiful young ladies.

I am no angel, neither am I a miracle boy nor Australia's favourite son for I am only as good as what I did yesterday. I will admit to being a dreamer yet I'm not the only one. The trouble with dreams, though, is that you have to wake up and do something about them. For many years I lived on visions to break the monotony of restrictions. When nobody could get in and I couldn't get out I used to imagine that I was one of my heroes, usually the champions of rugby league and cricket as I wanted to be just like my idols who taught me so much. When they were on the television my eyes were glued to the set and one day I realised that already I was similar to them. I'd fail in my attempts to break free if my emotions got in the way. When I set my goals, no matter how much I wanted to do things for other people it wouldn't work unless I wanted to do it for myself first.

Kerry Boustead, former Australian Rugby League wing, taught me one of the most important lessons and that was to feel good about myself and the effort that I'd put in, but above all not to let the pressures get me down because I wouldn't always be successful nor able to perform at full potential — although I could have a great time discovering the joys of teamwork. Kerry and his unpretentious ways help me keep my feet on the ground, and he is one person I wish I could be. His wife Leigh and their four children Lauren, Amber, Nicholas and Lachlan are the picture of complete happiness for their love binds them together to enjoy each passing day. The friendship they've given me has helped turn my dreams into reality. I count my blessings for having them in my life.

Every team taught me something and helped me look forward to tomorrow, especially during the grind of therapy. Then I would draw them close and be one with them; and grit my teeth and remember that however many knocks I had taken I had to bounce back to give it another go.

The Make-a-Wish Foundation helped me forget my life-threatening illness for a while and gave me one of the best weeks of my life by granting my wish to attend the State of Origin series. I rubbed shoulders with the men who play the greatest game of all. On or off the field they are simply the best bunch of guys. Their exteriors are as hard as nails but they've got it where it counts for they all went out of their way just to see me smile. May they, together with Ken and Mark

Arthurson, know that when they look at a blank face which cannot utter thanks, please take it from me that the heart is swelling with pride and the adrenalin pumping nearly makes me want to burst. To all who made that week possible and also gave my brother a night of glory, may you have all your wishes granted, too. You'll forever be in my thoughts and prayers.

If I should die tomorrow I'll wear a smile as I go for I've already had the honour of meeting the most awe-inspiring man I know — not because he is high on the list of Australia's greatest achievers whose deeds and music are full of wisdom and compassion, but because Angry Anderson is bigger than hate. It takes an almighty strength to love and give with total commitment the way Angry does. There is a place in heaven waiting for him along with all the street kids who look up to that man of magnificent stature. I can only hope that I am worthy to meet them there as it is their attitude and courage that make the world a better place.

As a kid from the bush with very little education I've been

blessed to have so many impressive people touch my life. Former prime minister Bob Hawke left a massive mark on my character and welcomed me into his home as if I was a king. But he is the one wearing the crown and to me has been a jewel in that of Australia's. Whatever Bob touches will always turn to gold as his style is in a class of its own. The thing I admire the most about Bob is that he admits to his mistakes; he is a people's person who doesn't forget the little bloke, and in my book anyone who has a passion for sports and horseracing can't be that bad. I have the highest regard for the great lady behind the man, for Mrs Hawke has a lustre and elegance not often seen these days and it's so nice to know that we still have such strong-willed pioneers in our midst.

Steady Eddy is a soul mate who fills me with a burning desire to laugh my cares away. He is one of the finest things to ever come out of a wheelchair as his sense of humour has won the hearts of millions. I know that Steady will go on to bigger and better success. He has shown that disabled people have an identity with the ability to laugh at ourselves; we might look different but we have feelings and dreams, too. All peo-ple like Steady and I really want is the chance to be a friend.

Laurie De Cole of TV's 'E Street' fame is my bandana brother who gave up his leisure time for fund-raising — you can't get a better mate than that. His aura emits a calmness, and those who meet him are full of compliments for this man. I'm positive Ray Martin, Wayne Gardner, Pehl from Radio Freedom, Scott McCrae and Andrew Matters are from the very same mould, as they are all wonderful people to be around.

I'll forever be grateful for having known and worked with Jane Hansen, formerly of the TV show 'Hard Copy' but now spreading her enchanting charm at 'Real Life'. The manner in which she portrayed my script is beyond compare; Jane's genuine concern will always be the power behind her success.

Shanna Provost from *Conscious Living* magazine is also someone I've been very proud to know. She is always sincere and kind.

To all the celebrities and media personalities I've met, I want to say thank you for the dignified way you've treated me. It was a great consolation in my time of need. Thank you for sharing a part of your human tenderness with me. The television was my teacher when I was too ill to go to school and watching you all made me what I am today. I've listened to your music and messages and after hearing what you had to say I adopted some of your ways. I want to pay tribute to you for teaching me to be myself.

Pro Hart and his lovely Christian family showed me that life itself is an art form; the number of churches we attend or the number of bibles we read becomes meaningless if we don't use Christianity in our daily lives. I have only been inside God's earthly homes five times all told and have not as yet read His everlasting words, but I no longer feel ashamed of not know- ing the secrets of old for that won't stop me from believing and trusting in my one Lord, or saying that I do. I know I've got a lot of changes to make within myself but only I can do it; God can't do everything for me and I'm glad that He has given me every experience for I needed every one in order to grow. From now on whichever direction I take I'm going to trust that

God is working out in my life what I'm meant to have. Having the gentle hands of Fathers Taranto, Burns and Keith, my three wise friends, makes the task much easier. Never do they preach about their calling or their woes for they just come to visit to put a sparkle in my life and keep me on my toes. Through them I have found a form of inner calm as I know that they are a part of the same learning process. They don't pretend to be higher or lower than me and have helped me learn to love myself.

I once thought that I was an undeserving and imperfect challenge but everyone who loved me felt that I was worth fighting for. Our God and earth and all who exist are much more important, so let's not be weak and destroy the God-given gifts that we've all been entrusted with. I believe we can work together towards an everlasting peace on this earth. It is fast becoming clear through scriptures, predictions, readings, music, television, acts of aid abroad and everyday life that we all want harmony. We can put aside our fears and negativity and love and accept ourselves and each other as one.

I wrote this book with the hope that we all gain a better understanding of disabled and everyday lives. With God's help, this is a creation of words from the heart and memory which strives to bring more moral awareness and enhancement of human kindness through dignity and truth. I hope through this book to obtain funding for the technology which has enlightened the lives of others once trapped and helped them in their struggle. There are so many others yet to be led out of the darkness so that they can help themselves to the bounties of life. However, all bodies, regardless of colour, creed, race or form, are only a casing for the soul. The greatest gift of all is to give freely from the heart. If not for teachers like Kerry and Anne Dickson my world would still be silent, a charity would not exist and the inner desire to encourage others would not have been nurtured.

In telling my story I have relied on my own memories, on what my family and friends have told me, and on the wisdom of hindsight.

Part I

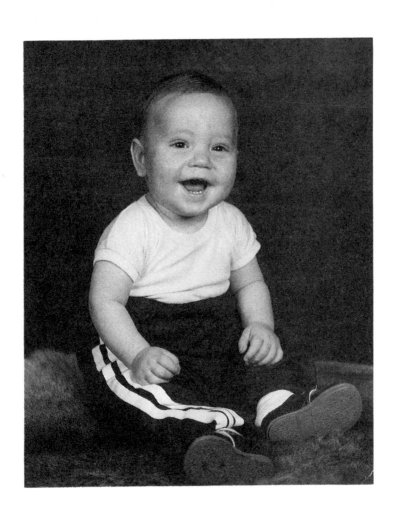

Previous page: Without a care in the world, four months before my illness.

Echoes from my past

Mother Nature spared me the torment of early memories of a normal life, that of mobility and speech with control over bodily functions. She washed away my memories of infancy, of being born a healthy baby to young but adoring parents, Sherron and Ian Harris, in September of 1977, at Gladstone on the central Queensland coast of Australia.

All traces of the illness which borrowed my wholeness when I was merely eleven months of age have been erased, as has the darkness of events during those bleak days of enduring gruelling treatments at hospitals. These cannot haunt me as they remain in oblivion. Also missing from my mental impressions are the drawn out hours of the coma I'd been lost in, along with any signs of hope in agonised eyes from my devoted family who gazed over me, whispering inspiration into my ears while surrounding me with faith that I would be restored to the original completeness of my birthright.

Left behind are the words of warning spoken by the doctors in charge of my case who sat on the fringe of an oxygen tent at my bedside, trying to prepare my grandparents, Campbell and Ena Gibbs, for the complications that may result if my will to survive was strong. Only time would tell if I'd weather the brunt of the disease which had them baffled. They didn't expect me to last the night and they felt that if by a miracle I did rebound it could be to a life of blindness and deafness or, in their terms, that of a totally dependent vegetable. However, it was never intended that their voices would reach me; the stark messages didn't become a part of my life. For I did rise from the coma unscathed, but only long enough to give my mother the last cuddle that I was ever able to; minutes later I crumbled in her arms as my once lively body turned into a physical wreck in front of their very eyes.

There have been various theories put forward as to the actual cause of my deformities. But it remains a mystery. It has been suggested that a mild gastric virus may have savagely attacked the cerebrum section of my brain, seriously affecting

4

muscle control and damaging co-ordination. I underwent many tests and suffered mild seizures. However, whether it was a virus, encephalitis or one of the number of lumbar punctures (a procedure used to test for meningitis) I received, there isn't anyone whom I blame for I believe it was just something that was meant to be. The doctors didn't maliciously set forth to cripple me thus I can't expect them to have done more than what they'd mastered at the time. They're not supreme beings who hold all the answers, nor can they perform supernatural feats — after all, they're only human and just as prone to mistakes as any person. All I can hope for is that some knowledge was gained from my situation which could help save someone else from a similar fate. I am but a speck as since the dawn of ages there have been multitudes of people who have inspired others by overcoming their challenges so that we can dwell in a better light. Their modesty keeps them from martyrdom and I'd shrivel at the thought of being compared to their valour as I will always pale in insignificance to them.

In my case it was an expensive lesson that many paid dearly

for in blood, sweat and tears. If my family had obtained compensation from a lawsuit it may well have defrayed the astronomical costs but it would not have recovered my body.

Through experience I've learnt that the best things in life are free and I'm already the richest boy alive because I'm loved and wanted. A healthy bank account may have eased the strains but even millionaires know problems and sabotage their lives. I'm neither scared nor ruled by wealth, for everything I've ever needed has been provided. I've come to see that when not used wisely or for good purposes money can give false power. But there is plenty to go around; those who have it deserve to be where they are or they would have lost it. However, I've never heard the jingle of coins tell me the words I am fortunate to hear from my family and friends who freely deliver their expressions of love and only expect a smile as their reward. They tell me how special I am to them, solely because I'm me, the person, not a poor little disabled urchin who stems from a working class background. My salts of the earth are my bounty which I'm more than proud to be a part of — anything else is a bonus as our simplistic lifestyle suits me because it mostly goes hand in hand with contentment. We might not have a hundred dollars in the bank or live in constant harmony but we're always there for one another.

Inevitably, medical equipment advances as does human knowledge but back then it was almost as ancient as some of the attitudes relating to what disabled people were and where they belonged. Nevertheless, in my opinion we're all handi-capped to some degree until awareness dawns and shifts the blindness of ignorance. If I'd been the way I am fifty years earlier they would have probably tried to lock the door and throw away the key. Even in my time old beliefs still stood, but thankfully I was saved from the discomfort of hearing crude suggestions by those who said that I was a useless piece of meat who should be hidden away and forgotten. I can't bring myself to detest them for expressing their grief in the only fashion they knew. Clearly to me they weren't aware that God doesn't create trash, only innocent children who grow up to be conditioned to think a particular way by other victims who don't know better. I'm certain they loved me in their own peculiar way but they couldn't possibly give me what they've never been shown themselves.

Untold times I've put myself in my family's shoes, endeavouring to perceive what they've endured by going through the paces of my transformation. They deal with problems when they arise and never complain; instead they hide their heartache exceptionally well behind a smile. Yet I only have to look into their eyes to see the masked pain and know that a part of them died when my freedom left. However, I don't have the sixth sense to begin to feel how devastated they must have been when atop of everything a specialist advised them to have me institutionalised because it was believed that I would never amount to anything and could only ruin many lives. I'm blessed to have an emotionally strong and close-knit family whose loving hearts and open minds made it possible for them to face such daunting prospects with unlimited vigour. They knew that when one door closes another opens.

My truest relationships were led by the maternal strength of my mother and the loyalty of her parents, Campbell and Ena Gibbs, and her brothers, Colin (Strop) and Robert Gibbs, which cemented an indomitable bond that has withstood the test of time. They allowed nothing to stand in their way in giving me a stable childhood. That alone is my greatest treasure which I cling to and cherish.

At barely eighteen years of age my mother had not seen a deformed person before, but she wasn't scared by my appearance or what lay ahead. Nor was she frightened of expressing her views; at five foot nothing she stood her ground and told the doctor that it would be over her dead body that she'd part with me. When it came to my welfare she knew exactly what she wanted and she wouldn't hear another word about giving me up. No matter what I looked like I was still a son to her who had grown in her cancer-tainted womb, a baby who she loved more than life itself and was far from being embarrassed over. My mother made sure the doctor heard her every word and, from knowing and loving my mum for so long, I'm certain Perth would have heard her, too. My uncles and grandparents fully supported her decision and became my towers of strength. They never once took a backward step where I was concerned, and their beautiful inner qualities blossomed. With all the grace and honest country values that is them they are true to themselves and don't pretend to be anything they're not. They are down to earth and rational people who would give anyone an even break. My family are straight down the line types who call a spade a spade and know what they want without going overboard. During the first really tough months all they concentrated on was my comfort and happiness. If my family had opted for relinquishment I would have had to accept that it was their choice and what they felt was best for everyone. I'm so relieved they decided to take a chance on me and I didn't have to overcome any added mental anguish.

I am full of admiration for the everyday selfless sacrifices that my family make for me, yet they don't make me feel insecure about their offerings as it just flows naturally. They've given me their all and then dug deeper to find the reserves to give some more. It is my belief that unless someone has really experienced it, they cannot fully comprehend the demands of living with a disabled person; the twenty-four-hour day in and day out parenting, which can be made easier with a positive attitude, and the persistent outside influences that are a test of the strongest will. However, life is what you make of it and it is not as hopeless as it may seem. Our family shares many practical jokes and we live each day as if it was our last. My Grandma Ena sums it up beautifully by stating that people are only tools, just like teabags who don't know how strong they'll be until they're placed in hot water. Our situation couldn't be changed so my family made the most of a bad experience; they didn't have time on their hands to waste worrying over what they no longer had so instead they focused on ways to improve all our lives and muffled their crying in the privacy of their bedrooms, or cried on one another's shoulders when they felt the overwhelming need to shed their distress.

After weeks of havoc it must have been soothing for my

family to be back in the familiar sanctuary of their home, away from the starkness and sterilisation of the hospital. They did, however, leave with praise for the new breed of nurses and doctors who'd waive the regulations to work with them and make the whole experience less frightening. I was taken home to be wrapped in comforting arms, once a place of relaxation and merriment where a rainbow of bliss had hovered until a few short weeks earlier. But it could be rebuilt as no soul has known a spectrum without tears. All it would take was time. I'd been labelled as permanently disfigured and brain-dead and my family had been given no insights into how to nurture a disabled child or where to go for assistance. There wasn't an instruction manual compiled by professional advisers or past carers who could fill the gap or warn of hurdles. Organisations didn't beat down our door with moral or financial support as there wasn't a register of afflicted people and what benefits they were entitled to. No information advising people where they could seek help was readily available. Like many other families, mine was left to find resources themselves and learn by trial and error. Unfortunately, the situation for families such as mine hasn't changed that much over the years.

My family swatted away the mounting odds and fought against the tunnel vision of others. They did not seek pity, nor did they turn to convenient crutches such as sedatives or alcohol. They knew that they'd only wake up to find further problems awaiting them and that the ones they'd tried in vain to escape hadn't disappeared. A trip away from reality can bring short-term relief, but so does the natural high of sleep.

Realising the value of support from others, my family sought out families in similar situations. However, they seemed few and far between. Some who were contacted even blatantly denied being the guardians of a disabled person, and said that therefore they weren't able to assist. It was a great shame they couldn't accept the support offered.

On the whole, my family trusted their intuition which served them extremely well. I thrived on their compassion, which I won't ever misinterpret as a weakness for it was indeed their strength.

They became teachers of one another and learnt something new every day while continuing with their lives where they'd left off. From the beginning they were comfortable about my appearance and accepted me for who I was. They believed I should have as regular a life as possible and so I went out with the family just as any child would. My family weren't ashamed of me; they didn't see the disability, only the shimmerings of the real me. They were also sure that they were doing the right thing and only wanted me to enjoy life. They loved me as much as they knew how. My family weren't obsessed by my shortcomings and didn't feel defeated, nor did they give a damn about what mediocre people thought. They had their fears and at times the hurt was unbearable but they pitched in to do what needed to be done. On the rare occasions when there were reservations concerning my presence or envy shown over the unavoidable extra care and attention I received, the negativity wasn't fuelled but ignored, and my family went about their way of treating me in the manner they'd hope to be cared for if they were me. It cost them nothing to be kind and considerate for it didn't take a genius to tell them that what happened to me could befall anyone. All too often they'd seen other lives dramatically altered from car crashes, strokes or whatever. They wouldn't leave me when I needed them most for they'd had their share of hard knocks and knew how great it felt to have a helping hand with a slice of the unbeatable human touch.

While hidden beneath my innocence of youth I didn't realise that in choosing to keep me my family were willing to yield much of their life. They took each day as it came so that I could be happy and have every chance to be the best person I could be. All they wanted was for me to have an opportunity to reach my full potential at my own pace. When they grew dissatisfied with what was on offer they looked for something better or created their very own. I was their labour of love and it didn't matter one iota that their nights were spent sleeplessly walking the floor with me screaming in their arms or that their days were filled with endless tasks orientated around my comfort. Their resilience was the driving motivation that kept them going so that I could have a quality life, without being confined to dependency, as they knew I would get a thrill out of achieving the smallest of feats. My mother tended to me during the daylight hours while my grandparents and uncles worked awesome hours to help cover expenses. But at night they all took shifts to console my aching body and calm my rage of tears that must have been shed out of the frustration of not being able to do what had once been so effortless and natural. Just prior to the illness which struck with such a debilitating force, I'd been able to walk and utter a few babyish words. These gifts had been taken away so quickly. Although I don't remember any of the gruesome details, I must have been fighting violently for the existence of a past which was still etched in my mind.

To me what goes around comes around for my family's patience and tolerance paid off when they made a major breakthrough by making contact with a paediatrician by the name of Dr O'Duffy. I'm led to believe he is in the correct field to complement his disposition as he gave my family the breath of fresh air they'd been looking for. Dr O'Duffy was full of constructive ideas which eased their burdens and he steered them to a spastic centre where I could be assessed and hopefully receive therapy. I was classified as being a spastic quadriplegic which meant that my family could be given home programs. From the beginning, Grandma Ena, my mother and Grandfather Campbell had exercised and massaged my limbs so that the muscles would not waste away and to release the rigidity. If not for their foresight my condition would have deteriorated and I haven't stopped thanking them for their resourcefulness. Despite having ongoing meetings with specialists, no-one had given them specific therapy exercises to do with me. I think sometimes the carers of a disabled person have a deeper understanding of the needs of that person than do many professionals. The professionals, of course, have a lot to offer. When diplomas and dedication work together for the same objective and people listen to each other's views, it is amazing what communication can achieve. My family attracted many local skilled experts to their side whose nobility showed from their concern and interest. They often put their own hectic schedules on hold. Dr Diefenbach and Dr Howe tried to help in any way they could.

City doctors were often cautious. One prescribed anti-convulsant medication which decayed my baby teeth, a side-effect Mum was not told about. So Mum had our dentist Dr Wilson monitor the damage. No book or medical journal can teach the power of goodwill as some things cannot be perceived with the mind; they have to be understood by a special kind of heart.

None of the medications were working and I screamed non stop. About three months after my illness another stepping stone to better things came when my mother took me to be examined by a qualified chiropractor who found that my neck and hip were out of alignment, possibly the result of my being held down while the lumbar punctures were administered or blood samples taken.

After the manipulations much of my pain diminished and I slept like the baby that I was for the first time since the whole ordeal began.

My family of marvels with staying power to boot weren't shy in seeking out alternative treatments once they'd been fully convinced that conventional medicine wasn't working at the time. But they did inform their practitioners of their intentions to stay within the safety line — I wasn't their little guinea pig and they weren't the type to clutch at straws. They weighed the consequences before anyone ever laid a hand on me. It didn't matter how many university degrees were hanging on the wall for they knew that although most people were honest there were charlatans waiting to prey on desperate people who'd do anything to make their ailing child well.

(Seven years on from these events we met Dr Maurice McGree who is now our GP. His insight and caring is remarkable. For instance, he has found 'twin' medications for me which are far less expensive than the one favoured at the time but just as effective and with no worse side-effects. Maurice makes sure we always have the best and most convenient care and attention.)

So much had taken place before my life properly began, with 36 months of my existence hidden behind the curtains of childhood which crept open to let the cracks of the past in. Everything so far had had a purpose. I was on the verge of unearthing myself to find out why I'm here and to becoming a better person. I was more curious than before but not as receptive as I could be. Ahead of me was the unfolding of a glorious journey balanced by highs and lows. From the start it was an adventure to behold with no time for rehearsals or for a long time to recognise and savour the delights. I didn't suspect that much anguish lay ahead for me and I wasn't prepared for the pitfalls or how to react to them. In fact, I didn't even know my own name. But I know now that every step along the way, every experience, was essential to me eventually being able to rest and not wanting to avoid looking at myself face to face and within.

In a way it seemed cruel and unjust that I wasn't aware of my disability, yet life was merciful in other aspects as I'd been left the legacies of hearing, sight, smell and thankfully, thought, with a sense of humour that gave me the magic of laughter which became a cure in itself and the best medicine of all. I often feel that I suffer from the Cornflake syndrome as the simple things in life are often the best to me. For my benefit also engraved in the corners of my subconscious was a sense that there was something peculiar about who and what I was. This strange feeling lived in the pit of my stomach patiently biding its time, waiting to devour me with shock. Once the truth did take hold it devastated every fibre of my being.

It felt so eerie to stir from the slumber of youthful nothing-ness to be greeted by a living nightmare. The thin veil between pleasure and pain had not yet been lifted. Two birthdays had gone by and my mental vision was still clouded but soon enough I was to find that I had a gift of the ultra kind, something far greater than anything I could have ever desired by having the genes of a family who had the ability to cope by always looking on the bright side of life and never giving up hope.

As I retrace my life, for I must look back and see where I've been in order to know where I'm going, the furthest I can recollect was when I was almost three years of age. My first memory is a joyous one — witnessing my baby brother's initial steps. Although fleeting and brief, it remains vivid within my mind as it became the foundation of my determination to conquer and escape from my catacomb-like form. This happened after I was fully attuned once the shock waves had subsided. It was the first fight my brain had with my body. As fresh as yesterday the pictures float back of me cradled in my mother's arms as she rocked me to and fro. My father was standing opposite talking to his brother Neil who had his arm casually draped over my Great Aunt Ida's shoulders. I remember the feeling of excitement from the party atmosphere for it was Mum's twenty-first birthday celebration. Everywhere I looked I saw people having a wonderful time, their laughter drowning out the music. Like most youngsters I didn't know where to look next as I wasn't going to miss a trick. Someone in the crowd startled me by calling out to Uncle Strop, but they'd used the name Colin which was puzzling as I'd only known him by his nickname. The next thing I knew he'd grabbed hold of me to whiz me around the loungeroom in a loop-the-loop style of dance which had my head spinning and caused me to squeal with delight. After a few turns he swayed with dizziness before placing me back in Mum's fold. He proceeded to fall over in a clownish display to which I laughed out loud. Strop certainly knew his audience and sat up to look lovingly into my eyes. I thought then that he must have been easily pleased to get such pleasure out of seeing me smile; even though he was a rugged man his interior was marshmallow.

No sooner had my eyeballs stopped flickering and the butterflies in my stomach ceased to flutter when Grandfather Campbell stood to propose a toast and presented Mum with a large gift-wrapped parcel which contained a sewing machine. That gesture really brought the house down as sewing definitely wasn't Mum's forte. But she was a real trooper who could take a joke and laugh about herself. She admitted she couldn't sew to save herself and held up a pair of my father's trousers that she'd stitched together while attempting to take up the hems — one leg was cut off to fit a man the size of Merv Hughes while Alfie Langer would have been lucky to have his ankles covered by the other.

Grandma Ena lit the candles on the cake and I sat mesmerised by the flickering glow as the party faded into the distance and I became engrossed in my thoughts. My attention was held by thinking of my family's unique ways for I'd watched those familiar and dear to me all night and one aspect stood out above the rest; they enjoyed one another's company and their happy-go-lucky habits flourished with the good clean fun. While I sat there feeling sentimental, Grandfather came to sit beside me and commented that you could take the people out of the country but not the country out of the people. For ages I pondered over his phrase as I didn't know that they had moved from the small northern New South Wales town of Emmaville to Gladstone before I was even a twinkle in Mum's eye. Neither did I realise that Mum was spooning a foul concoction into my mouth until my taste buds jarred with revulsion as the sour liquid slid down my throat. In minutes I was drowsy and could feel my eyelids growing heavier.

Suddenly, Danny broke my sleep-induced state by clambering from his crawling position to stand and walk straight towards me. I got such a surprise that I let out a squeal which startled Mum. As soon as she saw where I was looking her hand jutted out to catch Danny, whose cheeky grin and chubby legs charged directly into our clutches. I was on top of the world and filled with pride for my brother and tried to reach down to congratulate him with a cuddle. But he was only in our grasp long enough for me to see the mischief in his eyes before he spun around to take off again, exploring his new-found skill. He fell over a number of times but got straight back up on unsteady legs to try again.

More than anything I wanted to run and join him and with all my boyish enthusiasm I could hardly contain my excitement. Hurriedly I squirmed to get off Mum's lap and yelled out to Danny to wait for me as I was coming too. He looked back over his shoulder as if beckoning me to follow and the glint in his eye dared me to catch him, which made me all the more emotionally stirred. But as hard as I tried to wriggle free I was not capable of budging. I arched my neck to look down and see what was holding me back but Mum's arm shielded the view. I could feel my legs pressed together and suddenly felt foolish for panicking when all that appeared to be halting me was crossed knees, I tried to untwine them but still they wouldn't move an inch. My restlessness began to turn to desperation but I kept stretching with all my might, trying to get my toes to reach the floor. Whatever I tried, nothing worked. I was so afraid of failing that the rising fear inside was suffocating, yet I didn't want to allow it to beat me so I continued to struggle with myself for what seemed like an eternity; but that only resulted in sweat beads stinging my eyes. The whole time my head throbbed from asking myself over and over again if someone was playing a terrible prank on me. The lonely wondering of what the hell was going on was so real and I turned to my mother seeking answers but she couldn't hear my cry for help because all that had escaped from my lips was a deafening garble that rang in my ears. I screamed at the top of my lungs but still I was ignored. With every ounce of energy I had left I gave an almighty lunge but instead of standing upright I flung backwards to stare straight into Mum's face. She looked down at me and wiped away the perspiration but nothing was removing the heaviness from my heart and although I was surrounded by people at that moment I'd never felt so alone and lost. The terror of not being heard or able to move made me feel as if I was stuck in limbo without control over anything, especially myself. I was that dumbstruck I didn't really know what to think for my mind told me that I could walk and talk yet something was stopping me and I didn't know what it was. My natural instincts compelled me to keep fighting but I only grew weaker and more miserable. This was such a simple task and a part of life and I repeatedly told myself that if Danny could do it then I would too. Every time I floundered I seemed to be overpowered by frustration which pushed me into the pits of feeling so useless. However, my nature wouldn't permit me to give up easily as there had to be a logical explanation. Time and time again my attempts were feeble but I'd reassure myself that the next one would be successful and urged my body to work and have the vital strength to carry on until satisfaction was mine. The sleeping pills looked like they were going to be the winner as I could feel them taking hold and sapping my energy. In a last ditch effort I gave everything I could summon from within so that I'd walk before the night was over. I cursed and implored for this to work but I only struggled and fought to no avail. As I sat there like a shag on a rock I broke down to cry bitter tears of utter defeat which racked my entire body. Just when I thought there weren't any tears left to shed I looked at the sorrow in Danny's face and a fresh wave of disappointment flooded over me. That was only one of the many nights that I cried myself to sleep only to wake up to a new day to find that nothing had changed.

In the days following I moved between depression and bewilderment, living a life of self-torture, a lonely seeker who pushed closer to the truth to find my own answers . Each day I regressed deeper within myself trying to fathom why I was suffering in silence and not getting through to people; why I wasn't able to fulfil my primal needs.

A day or so later Grandma Ena came to our modest little country home at Bororen to be the breath of fresh air I so badly needed. She has a way of making everything seem better than it actually is and at that time her presence pulled me from the depths of despair for at least a few hours. Danny and I were to be bundled into her car and taken back home to Gladstone while my parents made another of their frequent relocating trips. No sooner had we started to adapt to one place than my father grew disgruntled and we moved again.

His alternating employment was the reason for most of the uprooting but I sensed his motives were more complex as he seemed to be running from something. One minute I'd think it was responsibility and the next I felt it was me, but it never occurred to me that he may have been fleeing from himself. Late that afternoon while Mum was packing my uncles and our friends, the McCraes, came rushing in Grandma's door. They were visibly shaken and terribly upset and one of them explained that my father had tried to run my uncles and their mates over after a trivial mishap. I couldn't recall my father being a violent man or that his personality changed when he drank but apparently everyone else was aware of it. They raced to Bororen to protect my mother in case she was to be the brunt of his anger. It baffled me that she wasn't told of the incident and I was scared of what they were trying to spare her from and what was hidden from me as things weren't adding up. It seemed that everything in my life was sad and elusive. I was engulfed in confusion and it was too much for my young mind to comprehend and bear, with me sinking lower with each passing incident.

That very same afternoon while everyone pretended everything was hunky dory, the answers hit me like a ton of bricks. It was during a game of hide and seek. Led by the older children, Danny had waddled off to conceal himself under a bed. Grandma muttered the countdown, hollered out the call of 'Coming ready or not!' and with me in her arms we went in search of them. We entered every room until we came to hers where, on passing a full-length mirror, a grotesque image reflected back at me. Grandma sat down to catch her breath and as I stared at the disfigured monster a sickening realisation swept over me, for that twisted wreck peering at me was me. I couldn't believe it for it was totally opposite to the picture in my mind. Surely it was a mistake — I couldn't possibly be that pathetic figure. However, the longer I sat there the more hate and rejection surfaced, creating pure revulsion for what I saw. As I looked into my eyes for the very first time I could feel my spirit ebb away, tears brimmed in my eyes and rolled down my cheeks and I felt so cheated and deceived. I hated the world and everything in it and screamed for someone to get me out. I wanted to know why those lifeless appendages were attached so rigidly to my body, disobeying every command; even simple requests weren't heard and I wanted someone to explain what was happening to me. I could hear them all telling me they loved me but I wanted them to stop this nightmare. No one heard my pleas or knew my pain; with all the begging and pleading I still lay trapped in silence.

Thereafter I sank to the deepest depths of despondency. I felt so inferior and inadequate, and trusted nobody except my family and close friends. I cried at the drop of a hat and felt less human every day. I was oblivious to what was going on around me, I didn't care less if the world stood still for I felt that mine had ended anyway. If I wasn't disabled and had to be fed I doubt that I would have eaten for the food got stuck in my throat because I didn't want to swallow a thing, certainly not my lot in life. I wasn't interested in anything for I no longer had any self-worth and I couldn't even escape with sleep; that wasn't to be mine either. The normally placid dreams were interrupted by visions of the real life horror, with most nights spent retching my heart out after I'd woken myself from being physically ill. I was given some insight, if not more disheartenment, around that same time from my first memorable attendance at a spastic centre. I was three-and-a-half years old.

I distinctly recall staying overnight at my grandparents' home. This usually happened on weekends only. Grandma woke me early on that Tuesday morning, which was odd because normally they'd creep around the house so as not to disturb my rest. I felt an awful sensation that something horrible was about to take place. After I was bathed and dressed we set off. Grandma drove and chatted away to Mum, who was nursing me. Even though the tropical sun drenched my face with warmth, my insides were chilled to the core. A while later our car came to a halt outside a red brick building. Just looking at it sent shivers through me for it resembled a blazing square tomb. As I was carried closer I became more nervous and didn't want to go any further but I had no way of running or saying how I felt. When we entered the glass doors my breath was taken away by the frozen atmosphere that enveloped me. I kept stretching, trying to tell Grandma that I was frightened and wanted to leave, but we were ushered into a dim, greyish room by a cheerful receptionist. We were met by three strangers who in seconds stood over me intruding on my personal space. They talked over me and around me, even about me, but never to me, as if I didn't exist. Despite not getting a response, my family and friends still included me in their conversations but these people must have thought I was invisible or not worthy of recognition.

I was placed on a mat covering the cement floor which hurt my bony back. Nobody explained what was going on so I just lay there listening to my heart pounding as the tension mounted within. One of the strangers was busy talking to Mum while the other two came closer and closer, lurking dangerously near. Before I could blink they were upon me like

piranhas, pushing and twisting my arms and legs in every direction as if it was a frenzied attack. The pain that shot up my
spine was excruciating, with each robotic tug and pull after
that sending sharp electrical shocks along my spinal cord that
only ceased for a short moment when the pain rocketed into
my skull. I was screaming out in agony telling them to stop, but
they only roused at me for being a naughty boy. The more I
tried to struggle loose, the harder their grip became on my
form. As much as I could I tried to push away from them,
hoping to break their hold, but that just met with insults as they
told me I was being stupid. That remark infuriated me and I
spat out a filthy string of oaths specifically at them; I wasn't
going to lay there putting up with their punishment and
humiliation as nobody was going to force me to do anything I
didn't want to do, whether I was a cripple or not. One of
them snapped at me, telling me to stop my rot and I retaliated
by saying that they could poke and prod me all they liked but
they'd never break my spirit for it was mine and all that I had
left and they weren't going to have it as I'd fight for it every

inch of the way. They could rape my flesh but they couldn't take away my dignity.

I was so distraught by not knowing why they were performing those incredibly cruel acts on my frame or why Mum simply stood there watching their performance. Yet I could see that she was upset and sighed with relief when I heard her telling them that I'd had enough. It was hopeless trying to express my opinion about the therapy but I had plenty to protest about inwardly and in my rage it didn't matter that they hadn't heard me. As I sat there sobbing I thought that surely they could guess that I was hurting or at least to know that my throat was parched from crying in a room without air conditioning at the height of summer.

Mum sponged me down with a cool washer while giving me sips of water. One therapist coolly stated that my session wasn't over and that it must be completed. My mother replied that it was finished unless it could be carried out in fun, using a different approach, such as toys to entice my participation. They looked at her as if she'd smacked their faces, and to me she had, with the truth. But they went on to say that she was neurotic and had to come to terms with the fact that I was disabled, and that she'd have to conform to their standards of practice. Mum just shook her head and said that the dark ages had gone.

Two therapists left the room while the other one came to sit beside us. Mum explained that she didn't want to argue or work against them but rather join forces with them. Yet she wouldn't tolerate me being distressed as I could be gradually eased and encouraged into therapy. The therapist said it wouldn't work and Mum cut her off to ask her for documented proof that their style did. I put my spiteful thoughts in for good measure and told her that they could do what they liked to me but I wouldn't relish their ways as long as they forgot what it was like to be a frightened child, or the day I saw them in my shoes enduring the same treatment.

I wasn't mature enough or at peace with myself to see reason, and they didn't understand this. Neither did I — I was too full of hatred to give anyone an even break. At the time our worlds were so very wide apart and I thought they were self-righteous do-gooders who stuck to regulations that were set for the majority, not the individual whose parents' input meant bugger all to them. I didn't respect their intentions, I wanted to get better and help myself. In hindsight, I can see that they were professional and perhaps if we'd been more receptive to each other, things may have worked out better.

During the journey home I didn't pride myself on my abusive manner for instead of a pleasant farewell I yelled obscenities at them. I'm sure they must have been pleased to see the back of me. I didn't savour my first experience but I knew that it was necessary for more to follow. But I didn't want it to be always like that. Back at home I licked my wounds and mentally healed my aching body — every tendon felt stretched beyond imagination. It was wonderful to have my routine disrupted to soak in a hot tub and afterwards have my taut muscles rubbed.

All this was meaningless compared to the tension at home where a dark cloud hovered over us. The storm hit on my fourth birthday, of all things, striking my parents with sorrow and devastating both Danny and I. In my doomed with gloom period I didn't know that any day could be special if I wanted it to be. Earlier that day I'd had a party which Grandma and Uncle Robert had organised. They'd decorated the backyard with balloons and tables packed to the hilt with calories. Taking pride of place was a boat-shaped ice-cream cake that my uncle had scrimped and saved to buy. All our friends and their children were there and I sat watching them play while Grandma fed me cake as if she was a mother bird as I didn't have the motor skills to chew by myself. Funnily enough, I didn't feel bitter that I couldn't join in all the games because I got just as much enjoyment out of watching the others. It wasn't their fault that I couldn't partake — even if I was a regular child it would have still been impossible as I'd had an asthma attack, probably triggered by the therapy, some-thing that had never occurred before but all the dis-ease was starting to cause diseases.

A lady who I didn't recognise arrived late with her daughter. She wasn't seated barely five minutes before contemptuously asking Mum who had the smartest and most developed child now. Her snide remark brought gasps from everyone within earshot but Mum replied that she felt sorry for her little girl as she'd always be more handicapped than me while she was seen as being in a competition because she'd never win her mother's approval. Mum said that children's progress varies and they don't need a weight around their neck. I saw Mum take a deep breath and hold her pain for that moment, but not so my uncle who ran inside. Grandma followed, carrying me.

Uncle Robbie had tears streaming down his face and when he looked up at me he kept asking why it wasn't him that had been struck down instead of me. He choked out that he'd had a happy childhood while I'd had none at all, and he wouldn't wish my affliction on his worst enemy. Grandma placed me in my uncle's trembling arms and said that children like me were sent to teach love and understanding and would never be as callous as the lady outside, for through me Grandma asked my uncle to learn to love his enemies, then he'd have none. She whispered that life goes on and I'd be happy but people who were jealous would never have a kind word for anyone or feel elated about the good fortunes of others as they were selfish and wanted it all for themselves. After working weeks at odd jobs to pay for my party, Uncle Robbie was just a kid himself and his balloon had burst in seconds. But his wonderful deeds live on forever. Mum came in to tell him not to take any notice of small-minded people who fail to see even the goodness within themselves and that the lady had done us all a favour because we could deal with our anxiety without wanting to get even. Mum kissed him and me on the cheek before going out to rejoin the dwindling group but shot back at us that success is the best revenge.

My mood plummeted lower than ever and to make matters worse my father hadn't returned from work and I felt that he'd broken his promise to me that he'd be at my party. Lately he'd been seeking comfort with his mates at the pub, but that was the done thing because men weren't supposed to cry or show their emotions. They'd brag to their mates but never discuss their innermost feelings with the women who shared their bed. I'd grown to know that my parents had problems before my inclusion but because of the pressures highlighted by my presence, I harboured the guilt that I was making them drift further apart. I felt so terrible for doing that to them and prayed that my father would forgive me for being his beast of burden which I surmised made him do the things he did to Mum. At such a tender age you don't know much of anything except disturbing patterns that are confusing and many things get way out of perspective.

I did learn that there is no such thing as a bad person, just bad experiences which can lead to inexcusable actions and behaviour. At the time I was very much like my father; neither of us had any self-worth. I wasn't feeling good about myself but my father will always be good enough for me. I forgive him for not being the father I wanted him to be for when it's all said and done he is partially responsible for giving me the greatest gift of all, life. I will always love him for who he is, even though we were destined to follow separate paths.

During the days of my emotional roller-coaster ride my father wasn't to join me at my party and I left hoping that he'd come over to my grandparents' house to kiss me goodnight. I didn't need a present and I didn't care that his parents hadn't acknowledged me for all I wanted for my birthday was a few minutes with my dad. That's the night I discovered that I couldn't always have what I wanted whenever I wanted it. He didn't come but Mum did, covered in blood and bruises as water couldn't wash away the harshness of my father's knuckles. I felt it may as well have been my hand that struck her for I was the one who'd caused the stress that was too hard to handle; I gave them the problems that led to the senseless act of domestic violence.

As I lay helplessly looking at Mum's swollen face I asked her to lock me away as the doctors were right; it would be best if they forgot me. I couldn't stand seeing the damage I'd caused and I begged for my voice to work just once so she'd hear me and see common sense. Without me around they could have their life back and time for marriage guidance. I may as well have talked to a brick wall for my silent lips were falling on deaf ears. It was apparent that Mum didn't want me to see her condition but she took hold of me and said that she didn't bring her children into the world for this kind of life. She looked me straight in the eyes and said that she knew she couldn't replace my father but women don't have to tolerate that sort of treatment even if she'd in some way provoked him. Yet she wasn't going to cover up and make excuses for my father any more as this was the last time he'd ever lay a hand on her. She said we'd just outgrown that lifestyle and it was time for my dad to move on.

A policeman entered the room and, although she was embarrassed, Mum asked for me to be taken out as she didn't feel I should hear her statement. But I needed to and screamed to stay as it was the only way of understanding the past. Before starting Mum asked me to never detest my father simply because he had a chip on his shoulder as she just wasn't the right one who he loved enough to want to change, and that she had to clean up her act as well. After listening it was evident that my mother was being honest but lenient in defending Dad, considering the revelations, but she felt she owed him and us boys that much in making a clean break. She didn't want a nasty divorce but wanted to be fair by splitting everything down the middle, as she wasn't going to walk without taking her share.

The details were explicit but brief because police mediators intended heading to my home but waited for Mum so that Danny could be handed over into her custody until the sordid mess could be sorted out by the courts. I knew that, although inebriated, my father wouldn't harm his son; detaining him was only a bluff. When the police arrived he placed my petrified brother into our neighbour Ray Brodie's arms before showing the police where his sawn-off shotgun was hidden. It wasn't meant for use that night as it was a weapon solely for pig hunting.

Watching my father being led away tore me apart for I didn't know if I was ever going to see him again. I called out his name but my whimper faded as he was driven off. I felt divided between my parents but couldn't take sides as I loved them both so much. Right then I wanted to be strong for my mother's sake so I muffled my cries, but the hurt and shame in my eyes must have given me away for she told me not to worry as everything was going to be fine. I was going out of my mind with the sorrow that was locked up in my heart. I'll never forget the policeman who came over to me and crouched down to my level to say that many things in life aren't easy with some people having to work a little harder than the rest but he could see that I was a born survivor who'd look after myself and my Mum. He tousled my hair saying that things would be better in the morning. As he ambled away I imagined that he must see some shocking things in his line of duty but it hadn't hardened him for he still had the time for a little boy's pain. He must have got a great sense of satisfaction from his life-threatening profession. Grandfather Campbell had been a prison warden and I knew that the pay wasn't near enough compensation for the risks. Yet these men were two of the rarities who weren't concerned about money as long as they did their job well, and went out of their way to help the underdog. They didn't see them as lowly and had an understanding that most of the jails and streets are filled with people who haven't had a decent childhood.

We went home to go to bed but everyone was still shaken. Danny was the worst affected. He kept screaming out in his sleep so Grandma sat in a lounge chair pacifying him next to her chest while Mum gave me a warm cup of milk to relax me. When everything settled down a family discussion took place with my grandparents telling Mum that their home was ours and always would be and that they were prepared to help us in whatever way she liked. Just when they'd raised their own children and should have been taking time out for themselves, they became our steadying influence and set about giving Danny and I the best years of our life.

On passing, a friend saw our light on. He'd heard about the trouble as bad news travels fast in a relatively small city. He came to offer any assistance he could. The conversation led around to my father and the man said some pretty mean things to which Mum told him to stop as she wasn't going to stand for anyone putting him down as she didn't want Danny and

I growing up being resentful towards anyone, certainly not our dad. The man told her to wake up to herself as she was protecting and eating her heart out over a man who was unfaithful. I'd never seen Mum let her guard down before but in that instant I knew she died inside and that it would be a long time until she trusted another man. It was such a low blow for Mum to wear, especially then. I knew at that moment I had to keep my father in my heart and hold on to my memories for it was my parents' happiness that mattered most of all. But I also had to let go of the hope that their marriage would survive.

Morning light delivered the sight of Mum slinging my father's belongings into cases while he was occupied being raked over the coals in court. Afterwards he came to tell Mum that he wouldn't stand a chance of contesting custody of Danny and me. He said that he didn't want to anyhow for she was a good mother and we were better off with her. In a devil-may-care attitude Mum told him not to do her any favours but to count himself lucky that his clothes were intact. Somehow I think a few items might have felt the wrath of scissors and had a sleeve or three missing here and there. My father hadn't appeared just to explain what had happened. I knew he'd come to say goodbye; in my eyes it was only another chunk of heartbreak piercing my life.

When it came to the crunch my innards screamed for my father to stay. I felt everything could change, I was the one who should have been leaving but if he wanted me to stay I'd behave myself, I vowed I would. How I willed my father to read my eyes so he would know that I was pleading with him not to go even though deep down I knew he must. I just didn't want it to end the way it was in such an unresolved manner. I felt my dad would miss many great moments in Danny's life, with no regard to mine for what could I ever achieve.

It's never easy parting with someone you love, even in the best of circumstances. And I knew that all my father was taking with him was bitter memories. It seemed to me that our time together had been so futile. While my father's kiss lingered on my forehead as he walked away, I couldn't help but wonder if he had treasured each day with me in the same light as I did with him. I'd hoped so.

During the days when I harboured many emotional scars I took it personally how quickly I could be replaced. I felt that the tears I'd shed over my father were wasted as I didn't hear a solitary word from him. I had fallen into the rut of expecting too much from people.

Months later, like a blast from the past he breezed back into my life with his girlfriend. She wasn't a threat as I was pleased that Dad was pursuing his dreams, but what left a sour taste on my tongue was the fact that for some reason he dodged paying maintenance. It made me wonder how much I meant to him. My grandparents made sure Danny and I didn't go without but that's what really pushed me over the edge. I couldn't handle seeing my beloved Grandma working her fingers to the bone. The guilt from within my solitary world sent me into fits of rage with myself. As I slunk deeper I looked at my life and it terrified me. At four and a half years of age I'd seen enough. If this was existing I didn't want another part of it for everything I touched turned to misery. And so I planned my suicide.

In my deeply troubled state it seemed to be the only solution and, even though I knew it was wrong to want to take my own life, it was my easy way out. I needed to escape and give everyone their freedom as I'd seen enough pain slicing souls. My family's love was unconditional but love wasn't everything I needed in my life. Over the next few days I said my farewells and had everything planned right down to the minutest detail. I remember questioning my body, asking if it would fail me. The time had come. Grandma was manoeuvring the car around the corner, the window was down and the road had my name on it for this was the chance to stretch and jump from the car, to end the suffering. I pushed, and struggled with all my might but Mum's hold wouldn't set me free and instead she scolded me for stretching. I cried because I'd failed, not because of her words. I asked her for goodness' sake to let me go and do something right. Grandma's roar instantly brought me back to reality as I'd never heard her speak in that tone ever. I shuddered as she hit Mum hard on the side of the face while telling my mother never to speak to her innocent grandchild in those tones again. That was my turning point. A jolt of realisation hit me; I'd been self-centred and selfish. I'd hit rock bottom by being blinded by self-pity and vanity; I hadn't truly appreciated the affection and sacrifices as I'd only thought about myself. My family must have been going through hell but they weren't feeling sorry for themselves, instead they united and formed a special bond, cemented by sincerity and laughter. They never showed contempt but only love for me. No wonder I didn't achieve — I wasn't focusing on my true desires, only my limitations. I had dwelled on my handicaps, and when I took the time to sit back and take a good hard look at my circumstances, they didn't appear to be as bad as they'd seemed. It was just a muscle disorder, after all! But I swear, if Grandma sings 'You Are My Sunshine' to me one more time I *will* commit suicide.

Part 2

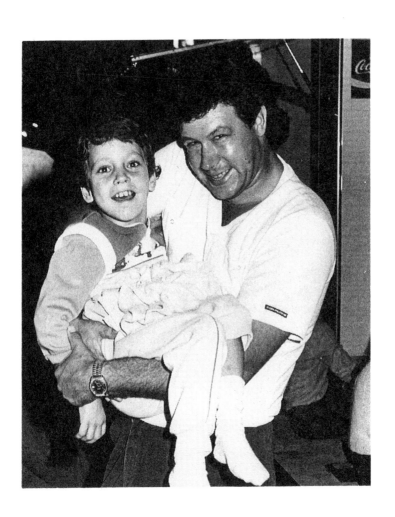

Previous page: What a relief! Home from Brisbane with my Dad, I never looked back. Everything happens for a reason.

I have a mind

On the dawn of my awakening my eyes were opened to the errors of my ways. In my weak-minded suicidal contemplations I'd held no regard for how betrayed my family would have been. I was only fooling myself by thinking that I'd be giving them a better lifestyle as the truth of the matter was that I would have left behind tortured and aching hearts. There and then I swore an oath that I'd try not to disappoint them or let myself sink that low again. I learnt a lot from toying with death. I had a better understanding of right and wrong, and I was beginning to see who I could be. I realised three main things. Firstly, that I had to stop taking life so seriously and forgive myself for my flaws. Once I could do this I could then accept others the way they are. Secondly, I must treasure every breath taken and cherish each moment with those whom I adored. Finally, I learnt that I must divorce myself from our judgemental society as I didn't have to be that way or believe the negativity in what people had to say. It was only their opinion and not my choice at all. Anything that was uttered I'd once taken to heart as being gospel without listening to what the inner me felt. I now realised that I had my own thoughts and beliefs. My family had shown this to me by never condemning the person I was.

In the two years since my first recollection a lot of water had passed under the bridge and the many unpleasant events that took place left their scars. But every sorrow was my own downfall and anger was my worst enemy. It wasn't the nicest experience discovering my affliction or the hurt of adjusting to suffering in silence yet that wasn't the most damaging thing that could ever happen to me. Then came the endurance of painful therapy which I barely tolerated or conformed to. I didn't like being forced and told what to do while listening to conflicting views. Although that need not have been such a great disaster, it left its mark at the time. In the middle of it all I didn't imagine that I'd ever get over my parents' separation and the violence which I detested. However, I did, as time heals the deepest wounds and love does conquer all. I just didn't have a dream that would take my mind away from the guilt of seeing my exhausted grandparents who I knew were working to keep me. I never saw the sign of victory, or at least not until I cleared the cobwebs from my mind. I looked at every interchange, wanting to comprehend what life was intent on teaching me, and heard my soul beating for escape to feel what human nature could do. The answer to the problems at hand came to me, for those who cared and gave did so by extending their love and expectations which was precisely the motivation that urged me to attempt to be that way as well. I'm still working on it.

The rivers of my mind were starting to flow freely and I sensed that I need do nothing but be my true self and happiness would follow. I had learnt by now to live with my disability. I could no longer afford to get involved in the games some people play if I hoped to put more joy and laughter back in my life and appreciate the good in others. Meanwhile I did come to the conclusion that when people put me down they are actually scared themselves. Besides, who were they to set standards for me to abide by when on occasions they'd been hypocrites who didn't bat an eyelid over stabbing someone in the back. At five years of age I found that the most dominating people I encountered were driven solely by self-gain and I was mortified that they never reached into their pockets or gave a thought to those less fortunate unless they got something out of it themselves. But it was senseless worrying so much. I felt that God would take care of their critical ways as a day would come when they'd need comfort too.

I'd been the one destroying my life and had many adjustments to make in only thinking with a pure mind and to stop being my own enemy. As I started afresh on the road to new horizons it was consoling to know that my will was still intact. I'd gained some insight and possibly a little pluck because I was steadfast that I wasn't going to allow the past to hurt me any more. In having an improved vision of life it came as second nature to know that there was bound to be a share of ups and downs yet I felt secure in knowing that every barrier I overcame would lead to better things. I wanted success without treading on anyone along the way and as I gradually came to terms with myself I fathomed that the power to change was within and that the hardest thing to see was always right in front of me. Almost immediately my attitude became much brighter with nearly everything having new meaning which turned so many awkward situations around to really start working for me. When I awoke early feeling weary from the lack of sleep, which wasn't unusual, I simply told myself that it was going to be a beautiful day as the world was a wonderful place brimming with complimentary people who wanted to help me and that I would make people happy with my smile until I had the time to catch up on my rest. The results were astounding for that's exactly what happened and I won't ever forget the exhilaration of knowing that I could achieve something.

While always allowed the freedom to be a child, I'd grown up slightly and no longer depended on another for my happiness as only my thoughts could affect my mood and my life. It may have been mind over matter but I felt like a brand new person as it was time for me to take control of my own destiny. But in the back of my mind I knew that too much of anything was no good for anybody and that I had to do what my heart told me and what my conscience would permit.

Shortly thereafter another lesson came when an infrequent visitor, who always assumed that I was unfeeling, dropped by. Each time we met he said many hurtful things and on this day it was that I'd be better off dead and if he had a kid like me he'd disown it. Mum tore shreds off him in her protective way, but being a gentle and considerate person she conducted the dressing down in a fashion which didn't bring her to his level. He was sternly told that no child, who she saw as an angel on this earth, would desire to be raised by a black-hearted man who had a yellow spine.

Instead of feeling bitter I truly felt sympathy for the sad and resentful man as he was someone's son but possibly hadn't received the affection commanded as a child. In growing older he may have been afraid of getting his ego bruised so he put on a harsh facade. It was all familiar ground as he was just one of a number who saw disabled people as unintelligent. I know some of us are not Einsteins but the degree of knowledge is only an examination of how much we know and not what we are able to take in.

That night I made up a prayer to thank God for bringing this man into my life exactly the way he was, and to pray for him. Actually I finally understood what my great grandmother Jinny once said of remaining silent if a nice word could not cross the lips. His know-it-all and do-as-I-say tone taught me to know my place as a child or man who in many lifetimes would not gain all the answers as I wasn't even an expert on myself.

It was enriching looking at my own growth for I found it to be remarkable that for once words of revulsion hadn't stung. I knew that insensitive people were about to leave my life as I no longer wanted to draw them to my side. However, that is far from being a pardon for my many thoughtless deeds as I also had to question if any of his weaknesses were within me. I had to admit that from time to time there had been.

When this man closed our door, which turned out to be for the last time, I sent him my share of luck as I felt he was going to need it more than me. On his way out he muttered something brash to my Aboriginal friend. I'd never been more proud of anyone when Cassandra didn't stoop to retaliating to his racial slur for she was a bigger person than that and didn't give it any energy. He insulted her again and I protested but only went into a spasm. I didn't care what he said about me but it dug deep to hear rude remarks about family or friends. Cassandra, on the other hand, sarcastically told him that he was only saying those things just to make her feel good and that she hoped he had a lovely day. Her skin may have been black but she had a heart of gold. To me the only difference between any human being is in intelligence and ignorance.

Whether this man realised it or not, we'd served a purpose in each other's lives. It taught me that I did have a mind and had to live at peace with myself; my body was versatile and important even if I couldn't control my form. I may want to move my right side and my left responds, but after all it is only a casing for my soul. I was determined that my body would no longer manipulate my mind. That afternoon the opportunity arose for me to look back into Grandma's mirror and a wonderful thing happened. I found that I finally approved of myself. As I affirmed those words I felt a surge of self-respect and as soul-searching as it was, I knew there'd be no going back. I had every intention of utilising what remained of my brain.

There's no time like the present, so I immediately set about devising a 'yes' and 'no' communication system with my eyes to form a link with the world. I was five years old. A few months later Grandma Ena caught onto my scheme of forcing my eyes up for 'yes' and down for 'no', and from that moment on I went from strength to strength. Grandma was reserved at first and kept her suspicions to herself. She quizzed me, to which I'd reply with my eye signals. But it got the better of her and she disclosed to my mother what she thought she'd unearthed. Mum confessed that she'd had the same notion and had been testing me, getting positive results. I laughed out loud at both of them. They called me a clever little bugger and the success of breaking free, as minimal as it was, meant more to me than all the gold from Ballarat. It was the first time ever that I'd had a conversation with my family. Mum and Grandma couldn't contain their excitement nor could the rest of my family. That evening we gathered around the dinner table laughing and joking while they poked fun at me. Strop and Robbie ribbed me with their Aussie wit which had me in hysterics as they mimicked how I'd walk if that was the way I talked. Even if I wanted to I couldn't take offence at them as it was great to finally feel totally included and, for a welcome change, to make light of my handicaps.

Somehow by laughing at my misfortunes it seemed as if the weight of the world had been lifted from my shoulders and my handicaps didn't appear to be as horrific as before. I realised how limited my thinking had been — I'd been wasting time worrying over what I didn't have and couldn't do. My burdens had blocked my vision of what potential was

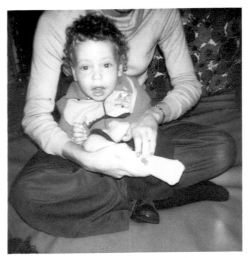

God, how I enjoyed therapy! When are we going to learn not to be afraid of change?

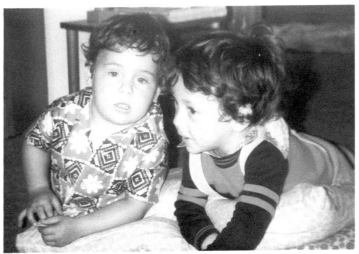

The wind beneath my wings: with my brother and hero, Danny.

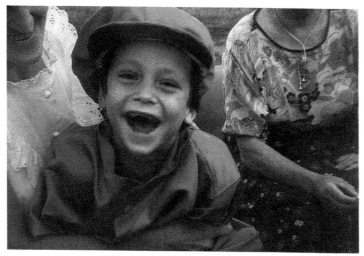

'Jim the Jockey' at the Gladstone Turf Club. Medication may have taken my teeth but I was, and still am, at the centre of my family's love and spontaneous thoughtfulness.

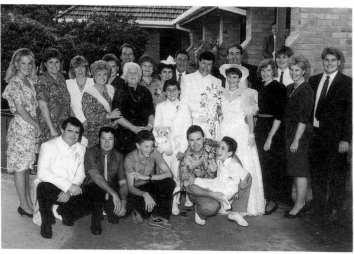

With some of the Gibbs' mob at Mum and Dad's wedding, one month before I communicated. I'd silently promised that I would sing at their wedding and I did—throughout the ceremony, the reception and all night long.

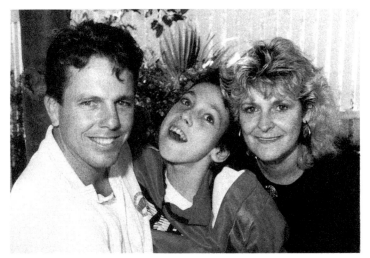

With two special friends, Kerry Boustead and Pam Provost, my guiding lights who share the fire in my heart for what Silence Isn't Golden represents.

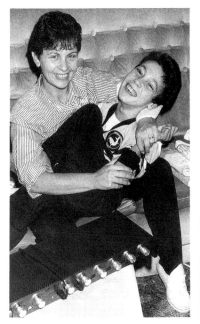

My only endorsement, the Unitems muscle stimulator. It is not the ultimate cure, but I and many others have had our lives turned around by the positive physical results of using this machine.

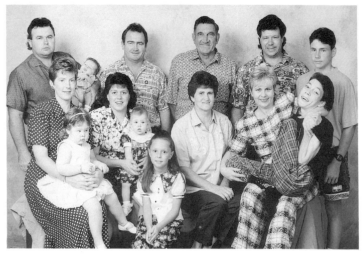

The power of love, my family, February 1994. Many are not in the photograph, but they continue to be the force in my life.

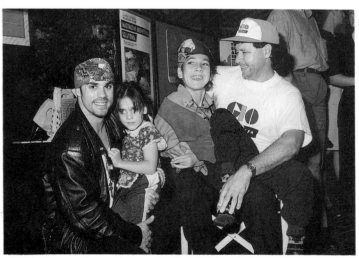

Dad and I with Kate Ferguson and my 'bandana brother', Laurie De'Cole. Kate squeezed my hand in thanks for her donated Unitems machine, a simple gesture that I will always treasure, although Pam Provost deserves all the credit.

untapped and I figured that life is too bountiful to be in opposition with myself all the time. The burning desire for knowledge had me wanting to live and to learn but especially to love. I was determined to gain wisdom if it was the last thing I ever did. I'd always possessed the ability to stretch in different ways for various needs, particularly if I didn't like a certain food or when I wanted to wrestle Grandfather Campbell, which was often the highlight of my day.

Mum and Grandma were very adept at reading my erratic movements, even when I misbehaved! They could double check that they understood my requests simply by asking me to look up or down. I took full advantage of my new situation and stretched when an educational program came on the television. It didn't take long for them to catch on so that I could select which show would assist me in my learning process. I had to begin somewhere so I chose 'Sesame Street' as my starting block. It became the teacher I didn't have. I'd memorise the shapes and sounds of the alphabet and then form words. But the English language was deceptive as the words weren't always spelt the way they sounded so I used other programs as my dictionary, usually game shows which consistently displayed data. I was forever seeking input and correction wherever I could find it. I was pleasantly surprised by how much information was aired daily and sometimes I had to take a break so that I wouldn't get confused. When I didn't concentrate on the picture many more new words leapt out at me and I grew accustomed to reading everything in sight, even biscuit boxes, road signs or cereal packets and whatever else I could lay my eyes on.

It was a slow and tedious method, but rewarding as I progressed from letters to words and then formed sentences. These were stored in my mind as if it was a computer for I couldn't manage pens and paper and just had to rely on brain power. In one way I was fortunate by being disabled as I didn't have the normal everyday distractions interrupting my learning, so I could easily centre my thoughts on the task and keep pushing myself further each day. I set my goals realistically so that I wouldn't find it daunting and want to give up.

Over the years I managed to gather a variety of valid word-age, but I believed it was far too restricting putting IQ before determination and learning from life, or the creativity that came from peeling back the pain. I learnt a lot from watching other people and at times knew what they were going to do before they did it; their actions or emotions said so much about them and even showed portions of their past. Life was where the real lessons were and my family and friends taught me much of what I know today. They were the reason and inspiration behind the poems I composed within my mind which stopped me from going insane.

On the rare occasions when my family ventured out with-out taking me along I was left in the care of either Grandma or Mum. That has always been the case as neither felt com-fortable about leaving me with anybody else. (Until recently a respite home didn't exist in Gladstone.) At times my mother dated but she wanted to give herself space without rushing into another relationship. At first it took a lot of coaxing to get her to mix socially again but now that I'm older I can relate to her caution regarding the dating game. In those days it wasn't the trend for ladies to be seen without an escort yet Mum and her friends Clare Briske and Anne Wreide weren't doing any harm. I was pleased that Mum was getting a release as single parents need an outlet too. In time Mum grew less bothered for she had the reassurance that Danny and I were having a ball in the more than capable hands of our grandparents. It came as a bit of a shock when she swayed in one night because we'd never seen her tipsy before. Mum did not usually consume alcohol and naturally a couple of glasses of wine at dinner went to her head. As we went to bed I got the giggles when she asked Grandma to stop the room from spinning and for days she was green. But she turned white a few days later when Grandma met her date at the door dressed in a bikini with a cigarette dangling out of her flapping gums where false teeth had once been, cold cream and mascara smeared over her face and curlers bouncing off the ten packets of bobby pins in her hair. The poor man nearly had a heart attack and when he looked in to see me he must have thought he was at a circus. What really made his eyes widen was Grandma's exclamation that if he wanted to take her daughter out he had to bed her first. Need I say we didn't see him for dust.

When my grandparents went out they left a note or told Mum where they could be reached in case of an emergency. One night Grandma had forgotten to do so and raced back cloaked in a dressing gown in the hope of fooling me as I always liked going with them. She spelt out to Mum where they'd be and I laughed because of course I understood and knew that they were going bowling. For a period after that incident they spelt backwards and I laughed at that, too. Ineffective as it may have been, it cemented their faith in my six-year-old intellect.

Mum wasn't a mind reader and didn't know how advanced I was. At times she took Danny and I to preschool. It was wonderful being around other children and sometimes their inquisitive minds had them asking the teacher all sorts of questions. They were never cruel as some adults could be for their innocence as yet hadn't been tainted by misinformed adults.

The children readily accepted Mum's explanations and afterwards the subject was forgotten. They went off in their carefree way to think of me as a natural part of life. It was amusing watching little children drag their parents by the hand to meet me, saying that I was just like them but couldn't walk or talk. Or I'd chuckle when they'd ask for a special pair of scissors just like the ones I used. Danny was forever the protective brother and as long as I live I'll never forget the day he left his friends in the activity corner to come and help me fingerpaint. He took hold of my twisted arm, gliding my hands across the paper to draw what we supposed was a happy face. Danny didn't care that I couldn't verbally respond for he rambled on telling me his most intimate secrets and fantasies. It was normal for him to hold up his hands and ask me to look at the right for yes and the left for no. When the drawing was completed he beckoned for the teacher and whispered in her ear. I didn't know why he was being rude but when I looked down to see what they'd written my heart skipped a beat; there in bold lettering was inscribed, 'To the best brother in the world'.

Most afternoons Mum carried me downstairs to my grand-parents' rumpus room which they'd converted into a therapy area. To spare Danny growing restless or feeling left out her friends Fran Caughey or Donna O'Dwyer took him on special outings of his own. Now and then, when he could, Uncle Strop helped with the home programs. Mum, Strop and Grandma Ena (when she wasn't out working) were my speech, occupational and physio therapists who tricked me into enjoy-ing the exercises. Often Mum showed me cards with shapes, colours or lettering on them, then she'd hold up two separate sheets asking me to look at a certain one and I'd move my head in the direction of my choice. Uncle Strop rewarded my efforts by cracking one of his many gags and once told me that I wouldn't be a kindergarten dropout like Danny, who'd more or less been expelled for swearing at the teacher who hadn't given him an ice-cream when all the other children received one. Danny hero worshipped our grandfather and uncles who'd become father figures to him. At times they let an odd word slip which Danny picked up — it was enough to make Kevin Bloody Wilson seem as meek as Mother Teresa! Mum wouldn't follow the teacher's suggestions that a good old-fashioned spanking could do the trick as she's never laid a hand on either of us. From her parents' guidance Mum felt that if she couldn't outsmart a four year old whose habits could be ignored as they would be outgrown, then she shouldn't have had children at all. Danny and I didn't get away with too much as Mum was strict and during a reprimand told us of her love and that the world would be more cruel. We knew her rules and how far she'd be pushed and even with me being disabled both Danny and I knew where we stood as punishment was the loss of privileges. Danny had only copied his peers, and really they should have been the ones getting their mouths washed out with soap. But in my opinion, if swearing is the worst thing they'll ever do then they won't end up too bad.

Instead of leaving me to hang around bored senseless in a standing frame waiting for my muscles to ache, Mum and Strop would divert my attention by marching me down the street all caliper clad to greet my grandfather, who'd drive me back home in his work ute. On the way we'd give cheek to his workmates over the CB radio. Thinking about it now I must have really trounced their eardrums, as Uncle Robbie, Sonya Wort and Dale Thompson's antics never failed to make me scream. They should have been on a stage, but the type with wheels that would carry them out of town.

When it rained and I couldn't go outside Mum kept me occupied by placing me in a frame which Grandma had designed specifically for me; we called it the judge's box. The alternative was lying face down on a slant board borrowed from the spastic centre. Whatever therapy was undertaken, my mind was never idle. Following professional advice, Mum kept me busy by covering my face, hands and legs with different textures, usually shaving cream or plasticine to keep my senses alive and develop tactile skills. This was fine for a while but after months of having stuff shoved on my face and various parts of my body it began to leave little credit for intelligence. Mum fathomed the fact that I wasn't a baby anymore so put aside the less stimulating therapy and introduced me to some of her ideas. While exercising my limbs she played music, which I absolutely got lost in. Or she talked to me, asking questions that I could answer with my yes or no system. We made a scrapbook using that method which took many hours to compile, but we virtually incorporated everything we did into that raggedy old book. I'd look at letters to spell out what I wanted noted. It's indescribable how terrific it felt to see some of my thoughts taking shape.

After much persuasion the spastic centre made their communication board for me; at first they had doubted that I had the faculties proclaimed. In all fairness it would have been difficult to accurately estimate my level when I was still protesting over their handling. After weeks of pleading one therapist agreed to Mum's invitation to assess me in my home environment. Although I was nervous I wasn't going to ruin the one chance that we'd all worked so hard for. I went through my paces and afterwards she apologised for disbelieving us and said that she'd file a report. She hoped that would mean

I was no longer held back. Some of her colleagues dismissed her claims. Who knows if they thought we'd put funny weed in her tea to distort her vision! Even when shown themselves, they still chose not to totally believe so I just chalked it up to experience. I could do nothing but accept that their minds were set. At least I had a few people on my side who knew that I had cerebral palsy, not Alzheimer's disease. Maybe it was a catch-22 situation where many humans suffer from 'old timer's disease'. In years to come I'll probably be looked upon as having that disease. Even great inventors throughout the ages have been seen as eccentric until their conceptions caught on so I didn't stand much of a chance of making ground and breaking free.

The finest of organisations are often divided and not always in agreement but I couldn't blame the system or begrudge the lack of finance available. At least they had a number of sincere employees among their ranks and time has a way of bringing out the truth. Sometimes their programs grew stale but I could help myself by entertaining my curiosity with mind games. A favourite was counting how many times my names appeared throughout the movie credits on TV. Mathematics wasn't a chore, in fact I adored the intriguing game and unless I thank God and genetics for my wisdom in that respect I can't explain the solutions that I can so readily visualise. Some may assume it's a gift that I see the answers to numerical problems but to be totally honest it might simply come from opening up the mind. I'm often incorrect, as I'm far from perfect, and at times my body betrays me especially when I try too hard as I go into a spasm. But practice makes perfect and watching ABC TV helped to fine tune some mental processes. They present many brilliant segments, which I happily absorbed, but too much of anything never worked for me and I've never been able to resist a comedy. So sometimes I'd stretch to watch one on the ABC or on another station. It was wonderful to lighten up.

It was around this time — I was now six-and-a-half years old — that I began listening to my body and mind. When I felt

I was lapsing back into over-extending my capabilities and needlessly punishing myself I'd call a halt with a scolding and tell myself that no person need suffer on this earth. I had my faults but knew if I wanted something badly enough I would be able to reach it. It might not happen overnight, but it would happen.

I learnt that I had to develop my other faculties to compensate for my disability. I was led by the example of a deaf friend of mine who had learnt to unleash any restrictions and develop her other senses.

Grandma had an uncanny knack of picking up on when I was disgruntled. Because she was often at work, she'd been removed just long enough to see that not all was in accord. She broached the subject of horse riding and swimming and I instantly looked up as confirmation. There were programs available but regional facilities were non-existent. Mum went to a few handicap support group meetings which were led by John Meldrum, a guidance officer. There was a committee comprised of a sprinkling of concerned parents who had banded together to help themselves and their charges. They had some wonderful ideas for local programs but needed numbers to get their plans off the ground. The organisation was given permission to use a hall for playgroups and to develop therapy sessions, if twelve names could be obtained. At the time there weren't a great many specialists in the area but the ones who were in Gladstone were willing to help. Penny Page, a local occupational therapist, was prepared to offer her expertise and the spastic centre pledged their staff to assist as well. It would have been for everyone's benefit and saved the 140-kilometre trip to Rockhampton (which wasn't quite far enough away to claim expenses) or travelling to Brisbane to receive updated treatments. It was costly to establishments and carers so having a centre in Gladstone would have been an ideal solution. Guardians had to take time off work at least once a month, not to mention the expenses of the trip, and I know of people who lost their jobs because of the many days away from the workforce. The list of our

needs is endless as there's always something new to be purchased and the cost of medication is always there. At present
I gratefully receive $102 per week from the handicap pension,
but some medicines cost $40 a week. However, the govern-
ment is like God and cannot provide everything, and it never
hurt anybody to try to better themselves. Some want to sit
back and wait for help to fall into their lap. Unfortunately this
was the case with some people in Gladstone and the self-help
group couldn't get the required number of people involved.
It was the same old cliché of not wanting to upset the apple
cart or admitting to being the carer of a disabled person.
Some people had regrets as their children had already moved
away from home into hostels, seeking professional help. So
the plans just had to be put on the scrapheap.

Grandma wouldn't be beaten and independently set about
taking me to my cousin Tony Gibbs' property or to Mr Jefferies
who lived down the road so that I could ride their horses. For
my seventh birthday my grandparents took on extra jobs and

bought me an above-ground pool. Years later, after much use and many replacement liners, which Grandma had also purchased, the sides of the pool began to buckle and rust away. Grandma got more than her money's worth, though, watching me exercise my limbs — half the time I didn't realise I was partaking in therapy as I was having endless hours of fun. When I couldn't swim in the old pool anymore the handicap association came to my rescue and donated another one. It was difficult juggling my pride but when I saw the pleasure they received in giving I truly appreciated the goodwill.

Each phase of my life has held infinite changes but one aspect remains paramount; being presented with every opportunity. Many options would not be possible without my family's ingenuity and encouragement to believe in myself.

We have conquered many battles yet the war of total independence is far from being won. During the merry-go-round of events which shaped my life I have tried to make the most of each day by physically and mentally working hard to capitalise on the motivation I consistently receive from family and friends. I've always been passionate about education as I believe in its importance. My motto to reach my ultimate goal of walking is to adapt and overcome.

I suspect there are numerous avenues that branch towards one ambition. In 1984 my mother announced to me that she was dissatisfied with the lack of professional interaction where I was concerned. She suggested we move to Brisbane. As my mother waited for my eye signal reply she went on to say that if we didn't explore full-time therapy we might regret it.

Where dreams are concerned hell or high water cannot deter me — some may see my stubborn streak as a fault but I know that nothing is impossible. Mum's words became a challenge yet we did not set off searching for miracles, although they are known to happen. I saw it as a chance to beat my fear of therapy. It was time for me to step out of the comfort zone; if I did not face the things that scared me I'd always be afraid of them.

Travel, accommodation and placement were arranged.

Nonetheless, we're a family unit and all needs have always been addressed. At that time Danny's needs took priority; he was a little boy, with thoughts and feelings, caught in the mayhem. When told of the shift, naturally my brother was devastated; after all, he was only five years old and it would mean leaving the only home he'd ever known. Grandma Ena and our Mum shared the same role as a mother figure, loving both Danny and I equally yet treating us as unique human beings with individual wants and needs. As young as Danny and I were, the past had effects, thankfully eased by untamed spirits and fires of the heart which separate them from sorrow. Danny chose to stay in Gladstone with Grandma Ena and, as difficult as it was, Mum and I headed for Brisbane.

We moved into a flat in the inner city of Brisbane. Our new neighbourhood was a culture shock; not that we are used to luxuries in Gladstone, but we certainly didn't have prostitutes, drug dealers and thugs living next door. However, we were near the centre I was to attend.

The very first day I greeted the teacher with a smile and, although I knew she couldn't hear me, I still said, 'Hi, I'm Bradley and I'll give you a chance if you give me one too'. I thought our new home was a shock, but it was nothing compared to the eye-opener I encountered in the very first minutes of entering my class. I'd never imagined or seen so many disabled people together — not that they were packed in like sardines, but I just didn't realise that cerebral palsy touched so many lives. I, for one, knew that it wasn't particular about who it chose for its next victim. I shared some wonderful experiences there and met some dedicated people who work tirelessly. I felt very humble around my classmates; for years I'd felt hard done by yet here there were people not only combatting a physical disability but blindness, deafness and torturous seizures as well — have you ever stopped to think that you rarely see a disabled person without a smile? The whole time I was there I was determined to make the most of it and there are only a few unpleasant memories, apart from the constant reminder that many don't know the love I have or a family as devoted as mine, a home of their own or even the pleasure of owning their very own toy.

It was the phase of my life where I discovered deep thought and reckoning, blocking out pain, tuning off when desired. Strenuous therapy was forgotten in dreams to escape the pain. As I stood tightly strapped, caliper-clad in the standing frame I often drifted off to faraway places; remembering, hoping, dreaming. I yearned for education but at that time I didn't realise that life was a very important teacher and that determination, willpower, self-esteem and outlook on life were the keys to learning. As I sat in the school bus looking at the people I'd wonder what made them who they were. Why were the unemployed sitting idly in the park when they could be volunteers at the centre? Why did the alcoholics give in to a bottle? So many thoughts but no answers. It was so frustrating at times. I had no control over anything, not even my body. I just had to make the most of my situation, without giving up. Every single day I missed my family but I knew I had to be strong — I had to try my best in the hope of making things better. Still I fretted and yearned for them. They were always a thought away, a happy reminder, the future, my inspiration, love and strength to do anything. Each day after school I'd stretch and arch my neck to check the postbox and I'd reread their letters a thousand times over. I'd pretend they were there and that we were happy and laughing.

There were times of welcome relief, such as trips to Emmaville. I remember fondly those nights around the piano with my great-grandmother Jinny (playing, and sometimes doing the Highland Fling), Laurie and Lola, Phoebe and Stan, Olga and Alan, Murphy and Pat, and the whole brood of children. We'd also go out to Rex and Eva's property at the nearby Gulf. Margaret and Ned, Kelvin and Gay, Dilly, Toddy and Alice, and all the kids would be there. We'd pitch tents in the yard and go cray-bobbing in the creek.

In the school holidays Mum and I would come home to Gladstone for a break. I rejoiced to be with my family again, to melt in Grandma's arms. It was on one of these trips that I met

Peter, now my dad, at a family party. I'd always had an uncanny knack of picking people, not judging but just seeing the goodness. I liked him in an instant and recall asking myself how I could get the message across to Mum that I approved. I stretched, trying to get closer, trying to get them together. Mum told me to sit up and behave myself but I ignored her and kept stretching until I got my way. I had to do something extraordinary — I wanted Peter to nurse me. It must have been hard for Mum to understand because I'd never sat with my uncles for a very long time let alone a stranger, but this was my way, my signal, Mum knew me so well. I know she must have been bewildered but it worked. Peter came to Brisbane often, bringing a welcome relief, adding sunshine to my life and to Mum's. Sometimes Grandma and Danny came too, and we had some fun times amidst the turmoil.

As I got to know Peter better I grew to admire his courage and strength, the gentle giant attitude; I'd look into his eyes and see kindness. It was easy to imagine us as a happy family. He always spoke to me, not at me, and I know he loved me for myself from the start. I wanted to be just like him when I grew up and that thought pulled me through many rough days.

There were times when I was outraged. I knew I was sick, tired and cranky and that there is good and bad in all of us and that I shouldn't take my frustrations out on others but sometimes it was hard to understand why some people were nasty, beyond the call of duty. I used to tell them sticks and stones or swear at them — I'm no angel. Each passing day my stomach burned, every morsel of food sent my stomach into a frenzy; I was often short-tempered. One particular day the bus driver shook me violently and threw me like a sack of potatoes onto a beanbag for vomiting on his shirt. He spat these venomous words at me: 'I'm sick of you spewing on me, you little idiot'. I spat these ones back at him: 'Yeah, and I'm sick of being sick and your driving stinks worse than my sick ever could'. Just then Mum walked in and, boy, did she let him have it. I was so proud of the stand she took for me. He was a big man but she soon cut him down to size.

That afternoon after school I returned home, with a new

driver of course, to find my Uncle Dilly (Harold) sitting there, so frail, a shell of the man I'd remembered. Cancer was ravaging his body but I never once heard him complain, never. He isn't alive today but I know he looks over me and knows of the courage he instilled in me.

I never thought I'd be indebted to a burglar but I am — because of him I was whisked back home to Gladstone by my knight in shining armour, Peter. Grandma has always been around to comfort me and this day she soothed both Mum and I and had us laughing even before we reached the outskirts of Brisbane. I whispered a silent prayer of thanks to the unknown intruder. I didn't feel like a failure for I knew that I'd given it my best shot, and I can't feel guilty about that. I settled back into family life and was at peace with myself.

I'll never forget the day Mum came through the door and announced that I'd be attending a normal school. My heart froze, I asked her if she'd gone bonkers — what was she up to now? As Peter carried me into the classroom my heart was beating loudly in my ears; I looked around searching for the cynics, the hecklers I'd imagined would be there. Instead I saw a wide-eyed woman trying to collect her composure. She spoke gently but clearly and gave me a warm reception. I liked her instantly, she saw the spark in my eye that I willed her to see, not the disability. How I wished to please her, this was a dream come true; I'd desired education for so long, my being ached with hope and exhilaration. I promised Anne Dickson that I would learn, reward her efforts with learning, push my mind and body to the limits. She gradually tested my knowledge and limitations. Anne made learning fun and I strived a little harder each time to please her — I would not fail. I was determined that I could do anything.

Anne fought for my rights as a scholar and explored every avenue imaginable. She touched on the idea of computers, arranging my introduction to technology. I'd tried to master a joystick at the centre without luck but technology had come a long way and before me lay the future. Anne tried me out on a communication board but no matter how hard I tried I failed; my body discarded the signals, every time I reached for the link my body rebelled. How I hurt that day. I'd failed but I knew Anne wasn't disappointed, that's the type of person she is. That didn't ease my pain but many things had built my inner strength and my mind knew the solution — I just had to get it out into the world. Every time I saw my communication board I'd stretch for it, slowly pointing, spelling each word, devising the keyboard of my dreams. The day my message ended and Mum relayed it to Anne I breathed a sigh of relief. It took six months to convey that message but not a second was wasted.

I attended school and loved it, the acceptance from my teacher and classmates was overwhelming. I will always be eternally grateful that they weren't blinded by ignorance. It was a great thrill that the kids would cheat from my eyes for the answers. How I loved those days, my teacher-aide Karen Leinster was always trying to trick me, unknowingly keeping my spirit alive for inside I was living a hell. The pain was intense, I'd block it out with happy memories, mostly about trips I'd had to Emmaville, my family there, of faraway places, recite the poetry I'd conjured in my mind, recall the times the people of

Gladstone had touched my life, my uncle's wedding, so many happy occasions, so many wonderful people, so many happy memories. Time ticked away and life went on. I was now twelve years old.

Suddenly one day it stopped — I died and experienced life after death. I'd never experienced such freedom and peace, such tranquil simplistic beauty, so divine, something to behold forever. I was whole. But I could not enter in, it wasn't my time. On my return I heard Mum say to Dad that she'd lost me and I said, 'Oh, no, you haven't'. Every day I'd sit and look heaven bound and say a little prayer of thanks for the deep understanding that lay trapped within me but sparkling through my eyes and smile.

I'd suffered the pain for years and conquered it with dreams. Every day of my life I was loved, accepted and taken to many splendid places. I'd drift into myself relishing my thoughts, on the boat, playing cricket and football or even at the races. Many people entered the lives of my family and mine, friends and relatives. Peter's family came to visit and I loved them as much as my blood relatives; they accepted me and knew that it was Peter's choice to be my dad. Every day the pain got increasingly worse and signs were showing on the outside. No matter how strong I tried to be, it struggled to free itself. My body shook uncontrollably with the pain, sweat beads stung my eyes; the scorching heat within the pit of my stomach slowly made its way up my throat only to gush back down to my stomach with ferocity, gripping, pulling, twisting and piercing my innards like red hot pins. I needed help — my eyes pleaded and begged for relief, my haunting screams were heard even though I tried to smother them. I tried to control the pain but it was unbearable and defeating. My family were going through torture watching me, trying to help, walking the floor, sitting on the edge of the bed trying to catch a wink of sleep.

Our family doctor was my eventual salvation. He initially transferred me to a specialist in Brisbane, but no matter how hard I try I can't forgive this man's uncaring, who-gives-a-stuff attitude. He wouldn't look into my eyes; in fact, he ignored me, spoke around me, and said Mum was neurotic in believing that I had intelligence. I'd often overheard Mum telling Grandma about the arguments she had had on this point but I'd never actually sat there and listened; I'd been spared that injustice. I asked the doctor as he gruffly pushed and poked at me if he spoke to his cat and dog and if so, how did he know they have intelligence? Of course he couldn't hear me but it was therapeutic to release the anger. I recaptured dignity when I met a doctor who stood firmly by his Hippocratic oath — Maurice McGree was caring, gentle and sincere, a doctor in every sense. He prescribed medication that relieved the pain and the suffering we'd all endured.

If only a tablet could take away the pain of the world. When you have love, health and happiness you're the richest person in the world. Nothing compares to the happiness that radiated the day Mum and Dad married. It was on the 29th of December 1990. I'd silently promised that I'd sing at their wedding and I did, all day, through the ceremony, while photos were taken, at the reception and all night long. Mum was so beautiful and happy; Dad beamed with pride. As I sat looking at my family and friends, new additions and old favourites, I counted my blessings for having the honour of knowing them. I didn't need a body — they were my pillars of strength, all cumulating to mould my being; my role models, the making of me. At one time or another they'd all formed a part of my body to make me whole, some my backbone, others my voice or arms and legs — they were all one big heart pulsating and pumping warmth, making life easier for me, creating dreams to always fall back on in times of need.

I'd certainly had a very rich, fulfilling, fortunate life, with the excitement of never knowing what lurked around the corner. I'd had another wonderful Christmas break and as usual it ended far too quickly but I was looking forward to my new term back at school. Beth, my teacher, always had a calming effect on me. She has an aura of serene beauty. On that hot January day in 1991 she asked if I'd like to try the new computer. As Dad slowly turned around and I glimpsed the object I couldn't believe my eyes. I went both numb and hysterical, a dream sitting right in front of me — dare I touch it? Confidence slowly built, fear and doubt — I experienced a million emotions in a few short seconds. I'd failed before, were my emotions strong enough to cope with failure again? This was my last chance, surely they'd give up on me if I disappointed them. Anne and her husband Kerry had put five long years into this, only to have their hopes dashed in a moment. Unfortunately they weren't there on this day for moral support. I couldn't disappoint so many people or myself. Flashbacks of my life passed before my eyes, giving me the strength and courage to at least try. I'd told myself countless times that I could do anything, I was alive, I'd be throwing away too much, I had nothing to lose and everything to gain. A tingling feeling rushed up my arm as I raised it, my mind was blank, Mum, Dad and Beth were busy talking; I wished for silence but they couldn't hear me. I was feeling guilty because Dad had been working long hours to pay for my medication, Grandma was at the farm slaving like a dog, everyone was working so hard. My determination grew like a raging fire. I knew I could do it and I kept repeating those words over and over in my mind with every letter I was determined to touch. The squeals broke my concentration, I looked at the screen to see if my imagination wasn't playing tricks on me, was I dreaming? No, no bloody way, I'd done it, I'd actually done it, I'd written my name! If the cow had jumped over the moon then my emotions were circling the orbit. Mum whispered in my ear to write something else — to coin a phrase I was dumbfounded and literally speechless, here I was out in the big, wide world and I didn't know what to say. So many things to say, I'd broken free, it felt so good, I was soaring, lifting to the highest of highs. I looked at the tears in Dad's eyes and told him something I'd yearned to tell him for years: 'I love you, Dad.'

I wanted to add 'with all my heart' but couldn't. I still wasn't sure of myself but I wasn't going to stop now, not when I'd just started. I pushed myself to write some more, to convince myself and add the confidence to do it over and over again, to grow stronger, to push myself to the limits, to work as hard as my family. I wanted to see that look of jubilation and pride on their faces forever.

I didn't want to leave my link with the world but I was exhausted and now was the time to relish in the celebrations. Every phone call brought new and greater highs. I realised that I'd tricked my body. It was over-confident in knowing that I'd failed before but I hadn't failed now, I'd won the battle. My brain beat my body or they'd relented and worked together. I don't know how the message got through and I don't care — all that mattered was the fact that I'd broken free, I could communicate.

When a computer donated by the Queensland Alumina Sports Club arrived, I wrote from the heart, releasing thirteen years of pent-up dreams and thanks. I grew stronger every day, able to say more and more. The sky's the limit, there's no stopping me now, and why should it stop others from having the same chances that I've been fortunate enough to have? We're human and live off dreams. It would be criminal of me not to help my friends, those still trapped in silence; they deserve the dignity to speak for themselves, they are individuals and have their different needs and desires. If it weren't for other disabled people paving an easier path for me to follow I may not have had the opportunities I've had.

I am proud of my feat, but I do feel sad that so many other disabled people who've broken free have not received the attention I have. Their achievements have been just as great, if not greater, than mine. And I know for a fact that some disabled people have given up hope of overcoming the barriers. I hope that by discovering that it can be done they'll give it another shot. The younger generation should be able to look forward to better opportunities. I decided there and then to set up a trust fund to buy much needed equipment for other disabled kids.

While I was in Sydney enjoying a week that the Make-a-Wish foundation had made possible I had another meeting with destiny when Pam Provost from Unitems strapped on a muscle-stimulating machine. This machine has given me the chance of a lifetime: the words from a doctor that I will take a step, I will walk and play the sport I love, run with my brother, walk proudly beside my loved ones, things I'd dreamed of forever. It's not a dream any more; it took my pain away at the very first treatment. I'd often wished for a massage and I'd pray that Mum's arm would stop aching from home therapy and nursing me. This is the future — technology is catching up with us.

Pam was like a breath of fresh air to me — she gets pleasure from giving, expects nothing in return, a smile of thanks is her reward. She works and gives from the heart, a rare quality. Pam's generosity has given me new direction and purpose for the future; many things would not be possible if not for her.

With the help of family and many friends, especially Pam, the Silence Isn't Golden charity was born. The first contributions came from all the wonderful people of Australia who sent me letters and money when my story hit the headlines.

During one of his visits Kerry Boustead learnt about my trust fund. He unselfishly donated his commission from the sales of

Unitems machines. In the meantime Pam set about raising more funds for Silence Isn't Golden.

While Pam and the others were busy making dreams come true by organising charity balls and the like, what could I do but dream and write, have fun and laugh, and be aware of what was going on around me.

I will never give up on my dreams, one of which is to set up a therapy centre in Noosa to cater for the minds, bodies and souls of disabled people. If I'm this happy for the rest of my life and surrounded by the ones I love so much then I will have achieved my life-long ambition. No matter what comes my way, I know I can rise above it and defeat the odds, and others can do it too. If we never give up, nothing's impossible. It's not the end, it's only the beginning.

Part 3

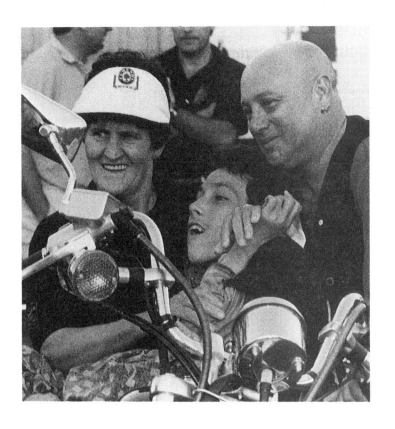

Previous page: Grandma Ena, Angry Anderson and I posing for the media during a Celebrity Bike Bash to raise money for Silence Isn't Golden.

To those special people in my life

I learnt more from my failures than I ever did from my successes. As much as I relished my home therapy programs with the volunteers, such as Leslie Skennerton and Mrs Howard, who occasionally helped Mum, what really spurred me on was enjoying the freedom of lying on a mattress in the loungeroom waiting with great anticipation for my family to come home. I'll never be ashamed that my forefathers dwelled in bark huts with dirt floors or were tin miners and shearers as they weren't afraid of hard work and earning an honest dollar. They hadn't lost sight of the true values of a close and loving family who shared the good times and the bad. They were bound to have their faults but all I've heard from people who knew them was that they were known to pull their weight and only ever offered friendship.

Apparently my family liked a good time but were one of the first to give as much as they could to comfort the needy and the poor, even though they themselves survived on rabbit stew. But whatever jingled in their pockets or was laid upon the table another was always welcome to share and no one was made to feel degraded by the deed. Some say they were humbled by the hospitality when they were told there was more than enough to go around. When they'd queried the fact that a large brood of mouths were to be fed, the answer came that it was easy to put another pot of water in the soup. From what I've been told of bygone days my family never put on airs and graces for they left the best impression by being themselves. What you saw was what you got. Their word was their honour and a handshake as solid as the ink on a contract. But God help anyone who abused their trust by stealing or lying; they gained nothing and lost a friend.

In my interpretation the next generation hasn't changed all that much. My Grandma Ena for starters adopted many of the Clifford and Purvis ways and is the mainstay that keeps our family together with her diplomatic and giving nature. She is just like her parents, Connie (née Purvis) and Edward Clifford, and I can depend on her being there through thick and thin with sound advice or a gentle hand that makes me feel as if there hadn't been a problem in the first place. She's told us all that there isn't anything that can't be sorted out but tell her a lie and we wouldn't sit down for a week. I couldn't count the times she's helped us all out and denied her own needs. Grandma's philosophy is to give now and not wait for some other time or opportunity. She doesn't take away my dignity and lets me 'stand on my own two feet'. All my darling Grandma has ever wanted is to carry on the tradition of a happy family who were comfortable going to her with troubles or triumphs any time of the day or night. My Grandma is as loyal as the day is long with eyes only for Grandfather. They've filled their home with love and laughter for family and friends alike. They don't try to keep up with the Joneses as they don't have a champagne taste with a beer pocket. Grandma sacrifices her sorrows and doesn't show many cares as long as we have a full stomach and are healthy and safe. She is the princess of practical jokes but isn't a drama queen for like thousands she grew up in the Depression and on the edge of war.

I may joke about Grandma's singing but many times she was the one consoling me during the dead of night. To some it would be natural to go to bed after climbing hectares upon hectares of mango trees in the tropical heat or cleaning houses or mowing lawns, but she chose to stay awake and spend precious moments with me. She's gone without countless hours of sleep to wipe my tepid brow when I was ill and racked with pain, then left for work at five in the morning and not returned until nine in the evening when she'd tackle the chores at home. During the solace of dawn my darling shared her thoughts or stories of old but never grumbled over parting with her wages for me. She is my strength that pulls me through. She knows I worry about her but she's told me that nobody was ever known to die from overworking or from a lack of sleep. I'd be rich if I had just one red cent for every time she's said that I'm her special angel yet Grandma is my saviour who I look up to with admiration and love more than I could ever say. She has the stamina to be envied by ten men whom she can outwork or swear with on the same par, but my Grandma is the most beautiful lady I know for her morals and ethics convey that God gave me one of the best. I'm more than proud to be her grandson.

I'm not going to wait until she's on her deathbed before I tell my Grandma that I love her and appreciate everything she's ever done. I intend making the most of the time we have now and when I have money she is never going to lift another finger again. Her stubborn streak will have her doing what she wants but someone has to be home to collect the little surprises I'm going to send. I won't wait until it's too late and end up putting flowers on her coffin.

I am one of the luckiest people alive to have Grandfather Campbell. He stems from the Gibbs and Brown clans who left the shores of Scotland and Ireland under the helm of our ancestors Sir Samuel and Lady Elizabeth Agnew. His parents Jinny and Robert Gibbs brought my grandfather Campbell into the world rather late in life, so he understood what it was like growing up with a father who was too old to play with him. My great-grandparents on both sides of my mother's family settled in the New England ranges where they made their mark. Edward Clifford for many years was the president of the Severn Shire Council whereas Robert Gibbs held the title to one of the wealthiest mines in the district until the Depression hit. As a lad Grandfather was known to be a larrikin yet wouldn't harm a fly and never killed an animal unless it was for food. He still has his love of the bush which he expresses in the self-taught piano wizardry that has enthralled me many a night. He composed a ballad for me and the words he sings of a mother's love with faith in God above could also relate to him. Grandfather has sung in bar-rooms and scratched tin to keep the pangs of hunger and cold at bay. All I've ever done was allow his Sunday morning stories to capture my imagination. Danny and I would cling to his every word and I could just picture the adventures in my mind. His tales of high sea piracy or winning the Melbourne Cup had Danny and me based as the main characters in the escapades. Our squeals of delight could be heard by our next-door neighbours, the Brodie bunch, and Jimmy, Sandra, Jason and Katie would yell out to turn the volume up so they could hear the stories too.

Grandfather has always been a worker but he took time out of his busy life to make my day just a bit brighter, whether it was an afternoon at the races watching my great uncle Kelvin's colt Boonanghi round the track (which set the stage for me being christened Jim the Jockey) or a fishing trip on Gladstone harbour aboard his boat when magical dolphins would steal my heart as they led our way. I'd sit on Mum's lap holding my line and waiting for a catch. Until recently I never knew that Grandfather always tied a fish onto the other end. He'd then sit back calmly watching the expression on my face as he snagged my line then jumped and hollered that I'd caught a bloody whopper. At times I thought I'd hooked a whale when he'd yell out to anchor his feet and cling onto our hats as he could feel himself being dragged into the depths. I got him back while playing cards, which we do most nights to see who has to do the washing up. It was purely accidental that I conveniently stretched back to see his hand and knew which move to make. As he headed for the kitchen I'd smile angelically at him.

In his heyday Grandfather Campbell once got six of the best on each hand from the headmaster's cane, then asked for more as they were pretty good. He was sent back to class with his mate to write an essay on cricket and scribbled 'Wet, no play', then recited a verse that goes: 'Dear Lord above, send down a dove with wings as sharp as razors to cut the throat of this old goat who keeps us here for ages'. Just last year his class held their reunion and many of his classmates went for the sole purpose of seeing how he turned out.

The hours I've spent with my Grandfather have been the richest of my time. I know what I'd like chiselled on his epitaph to immortalise my thanks for all the laughs. I can see the words of remembrance breaking the coldness of the grave to show what my grandfather was really like, a man who provided for his mother, wife, children and grandchildren with little thought for himself, so I'll use his own expression and say: 'Bugger the good looking ones, you'll do me'. When he grows old and the laugh lines fade into wrinkles I'll still be able to see the stories in his face. His body may slow in pace and his bones might creak from the days of carrying me but his eyes will always sparkle for he'll only ever be as old as he feels. I'll remind him of his words that the only thing in this life that we must do is die. When he does I know I'll surely cry for I will miss the magic of a wonderful grandfather's love. But I'll hear him calling my heart, telling me to keep my chin up. Then I suppose I'll hear his familiar laugh which I hold so dear and his words that the Creator whips him into shape with a flaming ten thousand volt lightning bolt. My grandfather is like his mother and would laugh at anything or do anything to make others laugh. He's already told me not to mourn but to celebrate because over the years we've had the time of our lives.

I have not been able to be a church goer so I don't know much about religious ways, but I talk to God often. I don't just call on Him when I'm feeling down for I like to give thanks for all the wonders that fill my day. Sometimes my heart grows heavy thinking of the many that haven't accepted God into their lives as all we have to do is ask and we will receive. I pray that in some small way I've given something back and it is my belief that God feels my gratitude and trust because He sent me to my Mum. I know I'm very lucky to have a caring and open relationship with my mother. I feel for the kids who don't have that figure in their lives. Many are caught in situations of domestic violence, alcoholism and drug abuse or sexual abuse, yet they run to their friends who, like me, think we know it all, instead of turning to a counsellor, teacher, family priest or kids' help line. They usually end up in further trouble. Appalling as it is, mere children are drug addicts, parents, prostitutes or join bizarre sects. I believe they're victims of victims who've buried their self-esteem and confidence. Thank God for responsible people like Angry Anderson who speak out and do something constructive in restoring the casualties of lost youth. When shown the way and that some moves were wrong, it's up to us to heal our own life. I greatly admire impressionable people who call a halt halfway through a destructive life filled with mistakes. By sharing how they've turned their life around it gives children hope to one day be the wise leaders and adults that we're meant to be.

As I rebelled I never gave a thought to the consequences further down the track. While feeling miserable I didn't see a way out and only attracted more havoc when there were people I could have listened to who were willing to help. I wasn't beyond repair or to blame for everything but I did have to accept responsibility and learn to forgive. My mother and I are very close but we don't have perfect rapport and at times we hold conflicting ideals. Although I couldn't answer back before I broke free, she dealt with issues fairly and calmly so I took heed of her point of view. I knew that no matter what I'd done she would be there for me to lean on. But what helped us the most was sharing mutual respect. I thought our love was worth fighting for even if it was hard bending both ways, but I didn't lose sight of the fact that she had spent hours in labour bringing me into the world. I figured she certainly wasn't attempting to wreck my life and was only trying to show me how to mend my ways. I also know Mum was young once and didn't want me to repeat her mistakes. Besides, I have enough errors of my own and it would be a shame to waste my life by not setting values for myself.

It might shock some that I wasn't completely wrapped in cotton wool to shield me from the world but what I encountered built my strength and insight and I learnt to appreciate and respect not only my beautiful mother but all women. She's always been there to catch me when I fall and honest enough to correct me when I stray. Mum has gone without and managed on a supporting parent's benefit or a meagre wage. It's been hard for her to make ends meet, but as far back as I can remember there hasn't been a day that I haven't been able to take the drugs prescribed to enhance my life.

Grandma and Mum made sure that Danny and I were always well groomed as they felt we could always afford to wash. When we were out they trusted us boys to be polite and use the manners which they'd taught us. Danny and I had nice clothes but around the house at times wore my cousins' hand-me-downs. As much as we would have liked designer brands Mum's budget didn't stretch that far and she hoped that advertising hype or peer pressure wouldn't be an influence or make us feel ashamed. We didn't worry because we had her love and other friends who also couldn't afford splashy shoes, and other mates who had no feet.

For sixteen years my mother has put her life on hold for me and many times she's been my voice. She got me to where I am today. To me Mum is everything that is kindness, beauty and gentleness yet she finds the courage to question con-formity. Whenever Mum is faced with an injustice which concerns us she's never afraid to speak her mind. Every day of my life Mum has been the one there for me. She practically nursed me in her arms for twenty hours at a stretch. The only people who have spared a true thought to her predicament are my grandparents who relieve the strain and take me to give Mum a rest. Mostly she is placid and likes nothing better than making me laugh, and I know she will defend Danny and I from the cradle to the grave. My mother has given her all and set her values high, and I couldn't think of a lovelier person who deserves to reach the sky. Good things come to those who wait and if I have anything to do with it she is going to have a life fit for a queen. I've never felt like a failure in her eyes as she congratulates everything I do.

In all those wonderful years together there hasn't been a day I wouldn't have given anything to thank her for being a special mum. She believes in me and every night as I drift off to sleep while lying on her weary arm, I hope that she feels the love that I am sending her in return. As the morning light shines upon her face I gently try to wake her with my smile to start her day as bright as she makes mine. Mum reminds me of wine; that lady who will always be in my heart just gets better with time. Never once has Mum pushed me further than I wanted to go, but the most important thing was that I should at least have a go. She's taught me to appreciate this land down under beneath the Southern Cross. I can sleep in peace without bombshells waking me, and I can go to hospitals that are comfortable and clean. I can eat food regularly and drink water as pure as rain and I can remember only pleasures and forget the dreaded pain. In a million years, though, I won't forget my Mum and what she means to me. I don't need fame or fortune as long as she is happy, even if that means being there with me. She's lived her life for Danny and I and along the way taught us about co-operation and what expectations she held. Having her backing I knew I couldn't go wrong for my mother has already made most of my dreams a reality.

In our home there are not many topics which haven't been discussed. It's wonderful listening to logic and hearing sound advice and knowing that my uncles are never too big to apologise. Strop (Colin) and Robert have set fine examples for me to follow as both have flown and both have faults. Although Strop's past 30 (and almost over the hill) he's still a big kid and often jumps in bed beside my grandparents to give them a hug and tell them about his day. Since being in the workforce

Strop has usually combined two lower paying jobs. When a commitment took him away from home I'd fret as I missed his enthusiasm and zest. When Grandma and Mum would take me to the park I'd sit on the old train and pretend I was visiting him. Grandma often carried me on her hip to walk miles across mudflats exploring every nook and cranny. Sea air bristled my nostrils and as I looked at the clouds I even pictured Uncle Strop there. On his return I used to think that all my Christmases had come at once for I had his ever-present smile close to me again. He'd tell me all the bulldust under the sun and I'd laugh at his tales until my sides were about to burst. I'm sure it was Strop who gave Danny the bright idea to play wars while on our treks with Grandma. If it wasn't for Mum disarming her problem child I'm certain Grandma and I would still be sitting on the crags ducking for cover as the little anklebiter bombarded us with rocks.

I could wrestle and box with Uncle Strop for hours and never once get hurt. Grandma supported me under the arms and he'd jab my sides with a straight left. I learnt to lift my knee to give him an upper cut. Grandfather was the referee and when we grew tired Strop would grab me as if I was a rag doll and we'd tackle Grandfather and put him in a headlock — we always got disqualified for interfering with the ref.

Strop must have spent a small fortune taking me for rides in his truck. If he bounced in the door asking how his little teddy bear was I knew that he was about to sweep me in his arms and in no time flat we'd be roaring down the road, the breeze parting my hair as Slim Dusty music blared. I'd sit up with my chest poked out as proud as I could be and look at my Uncle Strop who was just as proud of me. When he addressed me as Jim-Bob it was our signal that I was going to work with him and for ages I'd sit on his lap as he drove a dozer. He paid me by the hour but at day's end I had to shout him a beer because Uncle Strop taught me that that's what real mates are about. He said there's nothing wrong with helping someone out but a friend will forever pay their way or else they'll soon be known only as a bludger. Grandma taught us all that when we were guests we didn't have to go empty handed; whether we took drinks or a loaf of bread, something would always come in handy and be appreciated. We were expected to treat another's property with utmost respect and on leaving never walk out the door without thanking the hostess.

Strop might not be the romantic that I am but he has more principles in his little finger than a lot of men. He does have a drink and has done some wrong things but he's not one to argue or fight if he can help it. He would rather act the goat most of the day and night. I call him the Pied Piper to kids and animals for he has a way of drawing them to his side. I've heard it said that they know who to trust but Grandma would say that most children love a clown. Strop has had his share of problems but he doesn't make many of them known. He's shown me how to be an optimist and how to pick myself up with a funny thought when I'm feeling down. He helps me know the direction in which I want to go.

The city of Gladstone has always been good to me. The people I know don't treat me like a freak. For years people from all walks of life have stopped me in the street to inquire about my welfare — people such as Bill and Lorraine Geary, Beryl and Mackie, Fred and Pam Mason, and Jill and Graham Tresseder. The relaxed atmosphere and lovely people of Gladstone make it a pleasure to call home. My family and I rarely miss the annual show or Easter harbour festival as at each event we catch up with people we haven't seen in ages. Either Strop or Robert takes me on the rides, and they get as much fun out of watching me laugh as I do enjoying the amusements. My all-time favourite is the dodgem cars but it wouldn't be anything without the friendly people who attend. I find Gladstone to be a young person's city where the civic leaders encourage participation in sport and community pride. The industrial growth creates employment in this city which is the finishing line of the Brisbane to Gladstone yacht race and many times a Tidy Towns winner.

As a teenager my Uncle Robert had the opportunity to be a pro tennis player as his natural ability could be refined with the excellent coaches and facilities provided. His diverse talents allowed him to excel at many sports, including football and cricket as the competition was of a high standard. Good sportsmanship has always been the order of the day and every team member was encouraged to play for fun and not be downhearted if they didn't win. My Uncle Robert hung his twisted racket on the wall next to the array of trophies the day he threw it in a temper. (He was probably copying his idol, John McEnroe.) He looked up to see me watching and he felt so selfish because he could play and I couldn't even breathe properly. He said it was an infantile act and he was sorry that I'd witnessed it. But I didn't feel embarrassed by his behaviour. I personally feel it's better to let off steam, and he didn't harm anyone but himself.

Uncle Robbie's mate once referred to me as a 'spastic' and in no uncertain terms my uncle corrected him saying that I was just a little boy with a twisted frame who did not need a tag. Many times he's taken me in his arms to dance the night away or hold me as he's swung the cricket bat before carrying me to the other crease.

Like many Australian families, we've often played backyard clashes for the ashes. Just because I'm disabled it didn't mean that I had to sit and watch — I was always in the thick of it. I'd play for my birth state and the New South Wales mob would protest and ask me to undergo a drugs test which I never passed. When our new neighbour Mary Mastorini moved in she couldn't believe I was included in the games for she'd only known of disabled children who were placed in homes. At first I thought that in some way I'd upset her as she ran inside crying but later she told us that she thought it was so beautiful to see how I was treated. She does a wonderful job of it herself. Mary would do anything for me and she knows that I'd always be there for her. Uncle Robbie torments the life out of her but she takes it in her stride. He tells Mary that the ugly pills she takes are working overtime and that he's cleared a landing strip so that she won't crash her broom. I love sitting back listening to them share a joke.

Every other wonderful moment that I've been fortunate to spend with my Uncle Robert and our friends would fill ten books but nothing can replace our times at golf and home or where they've touched my heart.

Whatever else I've done I've always had my best mate at my side. If at times my brother Danny wasn't there in body, he always was in spirit. Although he hasn't taken a backseat or missed any pleasure that I've had, I admire him more than anyone because he's the exceptional person that he is. Danny has never once shown signs of jealousy and even at a very early age was more than understanding. I've been included in all his games and sometimes he torments me; my hero has done nothing but treat me normally. Up until the age of eight, every year he donned a Santa suit and rode in the back of Grandfather's ute, ringing a bell and throwing lollies to the other children in the neighbourhood. As he handed out our gifts he always kept his special present for me until last and I could bet a million dollars it was just what I wanted. Each year I willed for Mum to keep the tag attached for he is the gifted author in our family as what he writes comes straight from the heart.

When he was little he was a vagabond but his soul has always been as pure as falling snow. Even if Great Uncle Murphy and Aunty Pat gave him a chocolate his eyes would light up as if it was the most precious thing. As he grew older he loved me more each day and has never walked in the door without acknowledging me. He knew that I sat home most days as I was too ill to venture far. When I was at my worst he'd get up in the middle of the night and quietly check on me. I've lost count of the number of times Danny has fetched washers and whatever else was needed and not one single second did he whine. A lot of weekends he has worked alongside Grandma and isn't tight with his money. Danny has gone off on his own bat and brought me home the food he knew I liked or a shirt I'd had my eye on. He is undoubtedly one of the most thoughtful and unselfish people I know; a lad of fourteen who acts and thinks with more concern and maturity than many an acclaimed man.

Danny is pure class and likes the finest things in life but is prepared to put his brawn behind his dreams. There was an occasion when we were invited to go to the circus but the banks were closed and Mum only had enough money for the weekend. Danny didn't go off sulking because he couldn't have what he wanted, instead he showered then came out dressed with a fist full of notes saying that it was his treat and that we'd better hurry to get ready otherwise we'd miss the clowns. It is of no concern to me if I don't ever walk, for my brother makes me fly. It is an honour being near him and if I should die this day I've already seen paradise every time I look into his eyes.

Like many kids of today, I have two fathers and I love them both. Ian gave me life and he is my natural father. But, as Grandfather Campbell says: 'A lot of blokes can be a father but it takes a good man to be a dad'. For eleven years Peter has been my dad — and always will be.

My father Ian sometimes writes to me and sometimes visits. It's wonderful to be with him and see how we've both grown. It's a relief that there's no animosity or conflict between Ian and Peter.

Peter is my dad in every sense of the word. He is a tower

of strength to us all, a quiet achiever — his deeds speak volumes. He always puts his family first and his greatest satisfaction in life is caring for his family. He surprises us with his thoughtful gifts but the thing that really makes me laugh is his funny sayings. One of my favourites is: 'You're as handy as an ashtray on a motor bike'.

I sometimes feel embarrassed that people patronise Peter by saying he's a wonderful person for accepting the responsibility of caring for me, but I believe he deserves a VC and should be buried with military honours because he married Mum.

The following poem expresses some of my feelings about my fathers:

So many things I've never said
But I've stored them in my head
Lots of things I've wanted to say
Until the computer I had no way

Even though we're far apart

We're still in each other's heart

We have never tried to hide

Just what we feel deep inside

Although my body racks with pain

My love for you will always remain

Now I'm in my fourteenth year

I thought I'd get my butt into gear

To show the world that I am strong

Even if I'm different I still belong

That might be hard for some to swallow

For their souls are empty and hollow

But there's room for all to live

And lots of love for us to give

To let them know I'm a lucky lad

Who has a special, wonderful dad.

Part 4

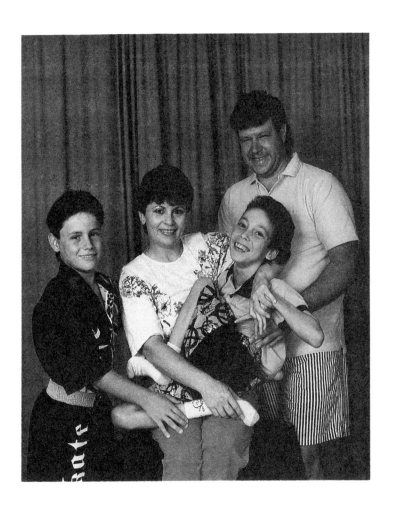

Previous page: The Wolf family — Danny, Sherron, Bradley and Peter.

Knowing Bradley

In the past sixteen years having Bradley as a brother I've never lacked love or ever missed out on anything. Although Bradley always got a lot of attention I could always understand and was never jealous or selfish to him for we both knew we loved each other. Before Bradley could communicate I thought life was very cruel for so many cerebral palsy children, not getting a chance to run around and enjoy themselves, until Bradley explained to us on his computer that that was the way of life and was meant to be, then all of a sudden I felt proud to have such a thoughtful brother.

When I was younger I always prayed that my brother would one day walk and talk. Although he had such little chance I'd always had faith and still do to this very day. I would some-times look in his eyes and wonder what he was thinking. When I look at Bradley I can't understand why he could be so happy for he has so little except love. I always try to imagine him walking around the room talking to us and wish it would have been me not him. Why him — of all the millions of people on earth, why him?

Daniel Harris Wolf

Someone once asked does Brad every play up — of course he does! To our family he is a quite normal sixteen-year-old boy and what boy up to sixteen years doesn't play up? He'll make loud noises when you want to hear something, he'll kick the table over (especially when there's an ashtray or drink on it), he'll spit his tucker out all over you and laugh about it.

To hear Brad laugh, I mean really laugh, is something that is hard to explain. His eyes light up and the deep cackle that he emits is something you have to hear to believe. He sort of makes everyone want to laugh and be happy. It's beautiful.

Grandfather Campbell

Words simply cannot describe how I feel about Bradley.

Grandma Ena

I attribute the peaceful look on Bradley's face to three things: the freedom of speech, the Unitems machine and the medication — and I couldn't ask for more. I feel blessed to have two wonderful sons.

Sherron Wolf

To have trusting eyes reach out and embrace in so many wonderful ways makes each day richer. Beauty indeed does come from within, pouring out, teaching me real courage, determination, diplomacy, patience, modesty and wisdom but, most of all, pride in being a dad. Knowing that my son suffers from nothing is my peace of mind and every reason to do better. It has not always been easy watching those eyes in pain and frustration or fearing they might not open by morning, but the fire in Bradley's heart and strength to smile through anything carries us all. To have the honour of 'I love you, dad' as his first printed words still makes me walk on air. Having confirmed by Bradley that his next breath is his greatest treasure is mine as well. I'm proud to have a son who accepts people for who they are while only seeing their goodness.

Peter Wolf

Someone once asked us whether we are ever ashamed of or become embarrassed with Bradley? I felt very sorry for that person. On the contrary, Bradley has brought more joy and love into our family than anyone could possibly imagine.

The love he pours out seems to rub off on everyone. We certainly have been blessed by having such a bright, intelligent fun-loving boy that words cannot describe. I only wish that a lot of other families had our closeness, then the world would be a better place.

Robert, Peta, Ashleigh & Blake Gibbs

We all knew what we wanted to say, but didn't know how to say it. Bradley makes many things look easy, especially loving him.

How do you thank someone for teaching so many lessons,

to let the world know just how blessed we are to have an unjudgemental and beautiful young man who has brought us closer, and makes the world a nicer place, simply with a smile.

'Strop', Sylvia, Rebecca & Taylah Gibbs

Your love and courage has been an inspiration to us all.

Ruby Wolf (Nanny)

Bradley affects people in many different ways. I observed a real rough, tough, hard drinking sleeper-cutter break down and cry after simply reading one of Bradley's poems.

Fame hasn't changed this young man one bit — he's still the same old Brad to me.

Graeme Wolf

Your sense of humour and affection has touched us all.

Gary, Linda, Toby & Benjamin Wolf

At first I was overwhelmed with sadness for Bradley — for the pain, frustation and humiliation he must constantly feel. But it wasn't long before I realised that Bradley would be very upset if he knew I was feeling this way. He doesn't pity himself and certainly doesn't want any pity from others.

Marie-Louise Taylor (Bradley's editor)

Part 5

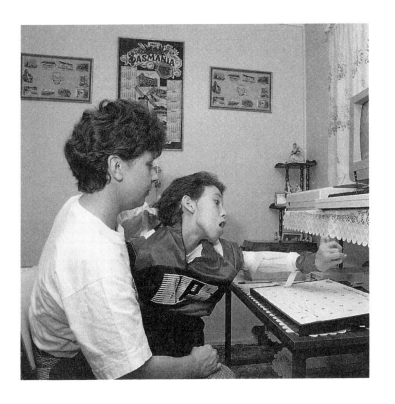

Previous page: After 13 years, finally I was able to communicate.

Breaking the Silence

Learning to listen:
Dr Maurice D. McGree

I first became aware of Bradley in early 1987. He was quite severely disabled and obviously suffered from cerebral palsy.

Cerebral palsy is a condition in which the brain makes messages to send to various muscle groups, including the voice box, but messages go the wrong way or sometimes don't arrive at all, so a person with mild cerebral palsy might only have a limp or moderate impairment of speech. The more severe the condition the less messages get through.

The degree of Bradley's cerebral palsy was profound. However, not as profound as his determination to cope with and overcome his disability.

It was evident that Bradley's mother and grandmother could communicate with Bradley. Simple questions such as 'Do you have a headache?' could easily be answered in the affirmative by looking at a light.

Mothers and grandmothers like Ena and Sherron no doubt began the art of healing. Over the millenia, patient observation plus trials of remedies led to a vast knowledge of signs and symptoms, names of disorders, as well as an armamentarium of medicines. Folk medicine was based on the knowledge of mothers and grandmothers. Their natural role as carers of the infant and child put them in this unique position of being the healers in the community. With the advent of a more structured society, the art of medicine was seized by universities. Learning became more formalised and healers even became known as doctors, in effect taking on the role of teachers.

I believe there is still a vast amount of observation being made by mothers and grandmothers. However, the traditional medical wisdom is that doctors are the fount of all knowledge and many no longer listen to mothers and grandmothers.

For a long time, Ena and Sherron have both had faith in Bradley's mental capacity. No one from the medical profession either heard the message or were particularly interested in making this observation themselves.

Thanks to Ena and Sherron, communication with Bradley was possible. He was therefore able to have input into his treatment and could indicate what his symptoms were.

It was very easy to build up a rapport with Bradley quickly and, even though he was often quite ill, it was evident that he had a great sense of humour and could communicate with others besides his mother and grandmother.

We always considered it necessary to treat Bradley as a person who required dignity, attention and had the ability to let us know his problems. It is very easy for a medical practitioner not to listen to an able-bodied person — so much easier is it then to be impatient and not understanding with a person such as Bradley. But with his quiet determination Bradley ensured that he was treated with dignity and respect.

Over the years Bradley has fallen in love with various receptionists and nurses, including Barbara Black, Stephanie Bates, Megan Kingston, Di Shore and, of course, my wife Jann. As soon as he was able to communicate with his computer he wrote a poem dedicated to them. As soon as it appeared, it was framed and it has been hanging in pride of place in our waiting room ever since.

My association with Bradley has been a humbling and learning experience. I am grateful for the opportunity to learn from Bradley, his mother, and his grandmother.

Bradley's contribution to us all is surely the art of communication. When he first looked at the light to imitate comprehension he brought light to all of us.

How Bradley found his voice:
Anne Dickson

In 1985 I was a Remedial Teacher (Learning Support Teacher) based at Gladstone West State School, a large primary school. My experience and expertise was in working with students with learning difficulties or learning disabilities and mild intellectual impairment. Of course, I'd seen some moderately and severely handicapped students in special schools, I had some theoretical knowledge about common handicapping conditions and I'd worked with students with a range of mild handicaps (including cerebral palsy) but had no first-hand experience of working with students with severe handicapping conditions.

One morning the District Special Services Officer, John Meldrum, came to talk to me about a young student who had been attending the spastic centre in Brisbane and who was coming home to Gladstone. John was familiar with the student's background and explained that although he was severely handicapped, entirely dependent on others for all his needs and unable to speak, his mother believed that her son was intelligent and she wanted him to attend a local primary school.

The student was, of course, Bradley Wolf. John said, 'I'd like you to read his file and consider working with him'. I read the file and my initial reaction was a mixture of emotions — shock, disbelief, sympathy and pure fear. I thought: 'This child is utterly dependent, he can't speak, can't stand, walk or sit unaided, has difficulty sitting in a wheelchair, has no control over gross or fine body movements — what can I teach him? How do I teach him? (Looking back I realise these were the wrong questions; now I'd ask 'What can be done to assist this child to learn?') John, in his wisdom, merely listened then said: 'Well, why don't you come with me to Brad's home and meet him before you decide'.

I remember our first meeting clearly — the twisted body, spasms causing arms and legs to fly in all directions, Brad's obvious delight at our visit expressed by gurgles, grunts and a range of facial expressions, but the most outstanding feature was his eyes and the intelligence and strong desire to communicate shining through. Our eyes met and at the same time there was a meeting of minds and hearts and our relationship was established. My fear changed to well, here's a beautiful human being with potential to learn, we'll find a way to help him learn. This was also my first meeting with Sherron, his mum — so young, nervous and anxious but obviously utterly committed to the welfare of her child and determined in her belief that his potential be realised.

We immediately began to plan for Bradley to attend school. There were many challenges to face — discussions with school administrators and teachers about reorganisation within the school to facilitate his attendance, how to transport him, what human and other resources were required to support him and, because of his frail physical state, what length of time was it possible for him to attend. With the goodwill of all involved, within a few weeks all was organised and Bradley began to attend school for just a few hours each week.

Before Bradley's arrival John and I had many discussions

about his program. We sought information from the range of professionals who'd been involved in his case in the past, but the most useful information came from his mother.

Three broad goals were set for his program:

- To provide opportunities for him to spend time with his peers.

- To establish a communication process with the long-term aim that Brad be able to instigate communication.

- To develop literacy: specifically, to teach him to read.

Looking back, I know that John and I had a strong belief that as well as providing opportunities for Brad to spend time with peers, there was a need for him to become as independent as possible and that this independence would be greatly enhanced if he could spend periods of time in his wheelchair. We also believed that communication would be established by the use of technology and that Brad would need to be in his wheelchair to access this technology. I'm not sure if Brad or his mum shared our goal of getting him into his wheelchair but at the time this seemed very important to us. (In the event, we were unsuccessful and did not achieve this goal.)

Our second goal was definitely shared by all. It was obvious that Brad struggled unceasingly to communicate with those around him and that his inability to communicate caused him enormous frustration. He brought with him a communication board with Makaton symbols (pictures of objects with the name written underneath). His mother was convinced that this was limiting and frustrating for him and she appeared to have no faith in its usefulness. It was immediately apparent to me that its usefulness was severely limited by his lack of control of hands and fingers to point to symbols.

I was strongly driven in my desire to achieve our third shared goal by my personal belief that if Brad could read, the world of books and ideas would be opened to him and his quality of life improved.

We did seek advice from a range of fellow professionals such as therapists and teachers at the spastic centre. The advice was undoubtedly theoretically sound but because my focus was probably more academic, there was little to help me with the actual hands on — the what do I do? — which was my immediate concern.

So Bradley started coming to school and working with me in a one-to-one situation. What *did* I do?

In the first few weeks a typical 'lesson' went like this: Brad would arrive and we'd spend time getting him into the wheelchair, a process which was obviously painful, uncomfortable and distressing, particularly as he often had chest infections and coughed and vomited frequently. Then we'd begin 'work'. Some days Brad would be too ill for this and we'd begin work immediately. If we had managed to get him into his wheelchair we'd work until his obvious distress prevented him from performing effectively before taking him out. He was usually in his wheelchair for only a short time, but we monitored the time, always attempting to increase it, but, as I explained earlier, this goal was eventually abandoned.

As Brad's only effective communication was by eye movement (and even that was often unreliable), all 'teaching' was done by giving choices. I'd write 'yes' on one hand and 'no' on the other so that he could indicate his response by looking at the appropriate hand.

Our 'work' consisted of working with texts so that reading skills could be developed. In the beginning I'd choose simple texts or I'd compose a text based on an experience he'd had which his mum would relate. I'd use the same approach that I'd use with any beginner reader: reading the text, modelling the reading process, discussing aspects of the text, making textual features explicit and discussing meanings and linking them to experiences. This is easy to do with students who respond physically and orally — looking, showing response with facial expression, pointing, talking, asking questions, offering comments, joining in reading and answering questions. It's much harder when you're limited to a yes or no response. I'd prepare special card material, providing alternatives, and use this in a 'sentence maker' (a simple board with pockets for inserting card material). In the beginning we worked with things like word/picture matching, changing letters, working

with phrases, re-ordering parts of sentences, sentence com-
pletions, matching beginnings and endings.

After a few weeks, when a routine and some workable
strategies had been established, a small group of students
joined Brad. At this stage his invaluable teacher-aide, Karen
Leinster, began to take over much of the one-to-one work.
She was to become a key link in enabling Brad to work in the
classroom. (When Karen left, Erin Boyle took over as
teacher-aide.)

It didn't take long for Brad to convince me that he could
read at least to the level of his age peers, and it was easier to
include him in literacy activities with his peers. He began to
have lessons in an ordinary classroom. We felt more relaxed
about his 'teaching' and accepted that Brad was learning by
being involved in classroom activities with other students.

Looking back, much of the early months was a learning time
for me rather than for Brad. We have a video of the early days
and I laugh now to think of how stupid Brad must have thought
I was asking him to match pictures and words when he was

already a fluent reader! The positive aspect of this early video is, I believe, that it clearly shows the expectations we had that he could learn and his positive response to our expectations. There's a classic illustration where he becomes distracted, spasms and loses his concentration. I, the teacher, pause and wait (impatiently) while his mother says, 'Stop your nonsense and get on with your work'.

With our confidence in his ability established and some workable strategies developed came the move to a classroom with age peers. One of the dedicated teachers at Gladstone West, Margaret Gibb, was working with a small class of students with special needs, some of whom were Brad's age peers. Margaret and her students willingly accepted Brad into their group. Margaret was just one of several dedicated staff from West who then and in subsequent years welcomed Brad with open hearts and minimum fuss. They include the principal, Kelly Hutchings (since retired), and teachers Peter Turich, Kym McAndrew, Keryn Potter, Jenny Lo Monaco and Gary Bolton. The model set by these adults and Brad's personality helped make it easy for fellow students to accept Brad and establish positive relationships with him.

This brief account makes it all seem a very smooth and simple process but, of course, there were challenges and frustrations on both sides. The main frustration for teachers was Brad's erratic attendance. He was often ill and would sometimes not be able to attend for weeks. Even when he did come to school, he would sometimes become ill during the lesson and he'd spasm so that his actual 'on-task' time was often just minutes. This meant that activities were often planned specifically for him and he'd be unable to attend, so continuity was really non-existent. His actual formal schooling has been minimal. I doubt that his total attendance and on-task time in the years at West would be greater than the equivalent of two to three full weeks of schooling.

Brad must also have experienced frustrations. He was obviously so bright. All teachers who worked with him tell of the times when the frustration of not being able to respond or to participate was expressed in actual pain, cries and almost tears from him. There are also many examples of incidents which convinced those working with him of his ability.

Brad left Gladstone West at the end of 1989 when he was aged twelve and enrolled at Gladstone Special School where my husband Kerry was principal.

As I mentioned earlier, from the beginning we believed that technology would enable Brad to communicate and we pursued this goal. I visited other educational facilities to look at the technology students were using and John was in constant contact with what was then the Technology Section of Special Education (now Adaptive Technology Services). Specialist staff from Brisbane visited us to assess Brad's needs and built different types of switches, constantly seeking some appropriate device, but it wasn't until that unforgettable day at Gladstone Special School that he successfully accessed the technology.

It was 29 January 1991 when the miracle occurred. Bradley wrote for the first time and his beautiful and brilliant mind showed itself to the world. My feelings at the time were joy and elation, pride but also relief — at last!

Of course what emerged was beyond my wildest imaginings — not only could he read and write, but the quality of his writing was absolutely outstanding. Even more amazing was his absolutely beautiful and complete human personality — he is accepting of his condition, is filled with the joy of life, has an engaging sense of humour (we always knew that!) and most amazingly lacks any of the feelings of anger, frustration or rage that could reasonably be expected. His absolute joy of life and the way he values the love of his family is an inspiration.

I've learned so much from Brad and his family and am always humbled when he says how much we've done for him as from my point of view it was simply providing support to a student and believing in him. Brad has taught me about:

- The indomitability of the human spirit. Brad's faith, determination and pure courage have overcome apparently insurmountable obstacles.

- The power of love. The love of Brad's family has supported and encouraged him and his own love of life and of his fellow humans is a driving force in his life.

- Myself as a person and as a teacher. My attitudes to handicapped persons and their parents and carers have changed dramatically and I hope this is reflected in the way in which I interact with them. As a teacher, I have learned many lessons and I believe there is at least a book to be written about implications for teachers and other professionals. Most important for teachers is, I believe, the message that attitude and acceptance are the most important attributes and certainly far more important than theoretical knowledge, a degree on the wall or any amount of skill. All of these contribute to the role of teacher but most important are basic attitudes of caring and acceptance.

Brad's story has much to teach us about teaching and learning and I hope that in time he will be able to help us explain his learning and unravel some of the mystery of how he became fully literate with virtually no formal teaching. How, for example, did he learn to spell without ever having worked through the stuctured phonics program that many people believe is essential and without ever having followed common practices such as learning five or ten spelling words every night and writing out the incorrect words five or ten times? How did he develop the vocabulary he has without having been exposed to this in his daily life? He gives us some tantalising glimpses. There is no doubt that television was a major influence. His family is not highly educated but he was surrounded by an extended family that used reading and writing to fulfil the real purposes of their lives and his extended family included him in all activities, constantly talking with him. His mother read to him, bought him children's books, made scrapbooks of postcards and news-paper cuttings and taught him about letters and words. His younger brother was observed doing homework and school activities such as projects. His grandfather composes his own songs and poems.

There are learning theories, particularly the theories of Whole Language and the Conditions of Learning articulated by the Australian educator, Brian Cambourne, which explain much about Brad's learning and it is one of my hopes that in time Brad will be able to fill some gaps and provide more insights into his learning as I believe his experience has many implications for all teachers.

He has also developed mathematics skills and can solve quite complex problems including those involving fractions, and no one has 'taught' him even basic facts. How did he learn these things?

If there is a negative side to Brad's success it is that it may have raised unrealistic expectations for some parents of the handicapped — that there's a mind like Brad's inside every handicapped child, just give them a computer and the same thing will happen. This is not necessarily so: just as within any group in the community — farmers or doctors, people with broken legs or black hair, those who drive red cars or are less than 160 centimetres tall — there is the full range of personality types and abilities. So within any group of people with labelled difference — autism or hearing impairment, spina bifida or elective mutism, cerebral palsy or Down's syndrome — there is a full range of personality types and abilities as well as needs and interests. Take any two people who carry any of these labels and they are different — just as you and I are different. So while Brad's story is an inspiration to all and has many lessons for carers and professionals working with the handi-capped, it is first and foremost the story of just one individual — Brad Wolf.

The concept keyboard

Brad uses a commercial model (BBC) of a concept keyboard. The concept keyboard is a highly sensitive touchpad which can be programmed in different configurations (e.g., in two sections to indicate two choices such as 'yes' or 'no', four sections, eight sections, and so on). Brad's keyboard is split into thirty-two squares with an alphabet overlay in A to Z configuration, basic punctuation and a delete function.

To touch the letter he wants, Brad makes a fist and the bone at the base of his thumb is the contact point.

His is an early model concept keyboard. Other more advanced and sophisticated models are now available and there is a wide range of other communication devices and equipment which are available to assist handicapped students.

In Queensland, the Low Incidence Support Centre pro-vides advice and information about technology for students with disabilities. The Regency Park Centre in Adelaide has been the source of invaluable information for Brad and his family. There are many other organisations across Australia, such as MACAS (Microcomputer and Communication Aids Service), which offer assistance and support. (Contact details for some of these services are listed under 'Support services: Where to start' at the end of the book.)

Silence Isn't Golden: Pam Provost

I met Bradley Wolf in 1991 after watching a television program about how he broke his silence after 13 years. When I saw how twisted his hand was I felt sure that the Unitems electronic muscle stimulator would help straighten his hand and make it easier for him to use the computer. I rang his mother, Sherron, and made an appointment to meet Bradley during his next visit to Sydney.

When I walked into the room and saw Bradley a bond happened immediately between us. Two weeks after Bradley returned to Gladstone, Sherron rang to tell me that he was able to hold a towel in his hand, something he had never been able to do before, and he had formed a biceps muscle. I flew to Gladstone immediately. I had seen amazing results in other children after using the Unitems machine and Bradley's response was major.

Bradley told me though his computer that the Unitems machine was the only form of therapy that he had accepted since leaving the spastic centre. He said: 'Get the message out — it works!'.

Bradley then asked me if I would be his voice and start a charity called 'Silence Isn't Golden' to help give his friends a better quality of life by providing them with much needed equipment like the Unitems machine. I was honoured that he had so much trust in me. When I saw the perspiration being mopped from his forehead and blood dripping from his mouth from the effort it takes him to write on the computer, I thought what he had asked me to do was minor.

Thus the Silence Isn't Golden foundation was born. One of its founding principles was to ensure that the administration costs were kept to a minimum so the money would go where it belongs — to the children. The foundation's aim is to buy Unitems machines, computers and other aids for children with disabilities that their families cannot afford. We are committed to taking a personal interest in each of the children we help and their families. We want them to look upon us as part of their family.

To start a charity was not as easy as I thought. We have had extremely tough times, but I have never considered giving up. The more Bradley's story was told, the more people would contact us for help. As the donations came in, every cent would go towards buying equipment. The company which supplies the Unitems machines, Hancotronic Australia, carried all the administration costs initially. But it is only a small company and after two years it had no more money to support the foundation. I put in my own money to help and I have worked for the foundation for no pay for the past three years but the reward of seeing how many people we have helped makes it all worthwhile.

I became extremely frustrated as more and more families who came to us for help told us the same stories: their children were not given enough therapy; they had to pay for the hire of equipment; and some were told that they should accept the fact that their child had cerebral palsy and no more could be done. Yet I was seeing with my own eyes the fabulous results of children having their own Unitems machine. For example, it made a dramatic difference to the life of Kate Ferguson, 4, of Landsborough in Queensland. Kate was facing the possibility of having her hamstrings cut to aid movement when her mother read Bradley's story and contacted us to try the machine. Eight weeks later, Kate's hamstrings had loosened and her back had straightened to the extent that her wheelchair needed adjusting. She took three steps and now she is crawling and pulling herself up. When I first met Kate she was like a rag doll, floppy all over.

Adrien Koutsou now sits up and people are asking if he is the same boy. Lisa Lehman had juvenile rheumatoid arthritis and wanted to commit suicide before she tried the Unitems machine. Now she is a driving force behind the foundation and has a great will to live. The treatment provided instant pain relief, more mobility and enabled her to hold onto things better by helping her to open her hand. Lisa had been facing the prospect of having the bones in her fingers broken in an attempt to improve movement, a move which could have ruined her future as a fashion designer. Now she is eager to get on with her life.

We have many more success stories like these to share and inspire us. Another source of inspiration has been Angry Anderson. Without the ongoing support of Angry, Bradley and the other kids, my family and loved ones, I would have given up long ago.

Without government funding, Silence Isn't Golden is struggling to survive. But it is still here, thanks to the support of organisations and individuals such as Telecom, Telecom MobileNet, Steve Grayson from the Gold Coast Harley Owners Club, the Lions Club, AustOtel Group hotels and celebrities such as Sophie Formica, Scott Wilkie, Nathan Harvey, Tony Bonner, Ingo Rademacher, Jon Bennett, Angry Anderson and many others who give their time freely for appearances at fund-raising functions and take a genuine interest in the foundation's work.

Our hard times have been outweighed by the good times. One of the most memorable was a trip to Bunbury in Perth to take Bradley out in the ocean to swim with the dolphins. We chose Bunbury because the dolphins there are not enticed in by fish. When we placed Bradley in the water, two dolphins swam straight up to him and in a matter of minutes the most amazing thing happened — dozens more dolphins appeared from nowhere and swam straight to him. Sherron and I just cried. When he came out of the water he was so relaxed that it was as if he had spent half an hour on the machine.

Often people ask me 'How's Bradley?' when he is there with me. I say: 'Don't ask me, ask him'. He is capable of answering for himself. This also happens to many of the other children with disabilities. My message is that if dolphins can go straight up to him so can humans. There is nothing to be scared of. He, too, has a brain and a sense of humour — let him use it.

Bradley has the ability to get to your heart like no one else can. At a ball we had for our 'Celebrity Bike Bash' fund raiser I was called on stage and Eden Gaha read a poem Bradley had written to me. The song he had them play for our dance was 'Wind Beneath My Wings'. I was overcome with emotion — there was not a dry eye in the house and Bradley was laughing.

Bradley Wolf and his friends have given me what no money on earth could buy: the feeling I get when a child develops a muscle, takes a step or sits up for the first time. I thank Bradley for giving me the chance to experience the satisfaction and inner peace this brings me. I also thank Bradley for his trust and belief in me and for guiding me to believe in myself. That honesty and dedication will bring the rewards of whatever he wishes to achieve. To the people who don't believe what's been happening with the children and in what I do, I urge you to take the time to see it for yourself and, with an open mind, you could feel the way we do at Silence Isn't Golden.

Our ultimate goal is to build a centre which has animals on the property so that when children arrive the first thing they will get involved with is nature. The therapy room would be painted in cool colours and the walls covered with positive messages from Bradley and other children. Both conventional and alternative therapy would be used and parents would have a major role in the running of the centre, social functions and other activities.

The Unitems machine

Electronic muscle stimulation, also known as 'electro-therapy', is a safe and effective way to stimulate and exercise muscles. Light electric current impulses, varying in length and frequency, are sent via electrode pads to the motor nerve fibres of the muscles. These impulses cause the muscle to contract and relax in a natural way. At the same time, the pain-sensitive nerve fibres are stimulated, providing relief from pain.

The rhythmic alternation between muscular contraction and relaxation increases the blood flow throughout the muscle tissue, exactly as it is increased during vigorous exercise but without the physical strain that weak joints and untrained muscles are unable to withstand. Using deep wave therapy, the Unitems therapeutic electro-muscle stimulator enhances circulation by dilating the blood vessels. It therefore speeds up the whole process of muscle recuperation well beyond traditional methods and is able to promote muscle growth as well as muscle repair.

The Unitems machine does in half an hour what would take carers hours to achieve. When muscles have wasted, it helps to build muscle bulk. For example, as a result of using the machine Bradley developed a biceps muscle and Kate's back muscles were built up to support her body weight. Her head control has therefore also improved considerably.

What is cerebral palsy?

The brain controls all that we do. Different parts of the brain control the movement of every muscle of the body. With cerebral palsy, there is damage to or lack of development in one or more of these areas of the brain. *Cerebral* refers to the brain; *palsy* means weakness or paralysis or lack of muscle control. The term 'cerebral palsy' therefore describes a collection of disorders which affect movement and posture.

Cerebral palsy affects the way people unconsciously organise a series of small movements into an endless variety of skills such as walking, sitting, eating, writing and speaking. However, no two people with cerebral palsy are affected in the same way.

Who has cerebral palsy?

One baby in every 400 born will develop cerebral palsy. There is no distinction of sex, race, maternal age or social background.

How is it caused?

The damage to the brain usually happens before, around or soon after the baby is born. Some causes of cerebral palsy are:

- exposure to certain infections in the early months of pregnancy;
- a difficult or premature birth;
- a serious infection in the first days or weeks following birth of the infant.

However, in many cases, the cause of cerebral palsy cannot be determined.

What are the main forms of cerebral palsy?

If you understand the different types of cerebral palsy, it is easier to appreciate a child's development and how that child will learn to move. There are three types of cerebral palsy: spastic, athetoid and ataxic. Many people with cerebral palsy have a combination of two or more types.

- *Spastic cerebral palsy:* People with this type of cerebral palsy have stiff or spastic muscles and find it difficult to move. Some muscles are tight and some muscles appear very weak. The part of the brain affected is the cortex. In spastic hemiplegia, the arm and leg on one side are affected. In spastic diplegia, the lower limbs are mainly affected. In spastic quadriplegia, the whole body of the child is affected — arms, legs and trunk.

- *Athetoid cerebral palsy:* People with this kind of cerebral palsy have muscles which change from floppy to tense. The arms and legs move a lot and the movement is difficult to control. Their speech is hard to understand because of difficulties controlling the movements of the tongue and breathing. In athetoid cerebral palsy, the middle part of the basal ganglia is affected.

- *Ataxic cerebral palsy:* People with this kind of cerebral palsy find it difficult to balance. When they walk, they are very unsteady. They often have shaky hand movements and jerky speech. Ataxic cerebral palsy is a result of damage to the cerebellum at the base of the brain.

What are the effects?

Children with cerebral palsy are delayed in the development of some or all of their milestones, such as sitting, standing and walking. Some with severe cerebral palsy may never master these milestones. As the child grows older, the degree of disability becomes clearer. Clumsiness in a toddler may be accepted as normal, whereas the same degree of clumsiness in a six year old is not.

For other children, once milestones are achieved they become automatic. So once a child is walking, he or she no longer needs to think about it — only where they are going and what they want to do when they get there.

For most children and adults with cerebral palsy, their movements and activities never become as automatic. For example, a child or adult whose walking is not automatic can walk while concentrating, but if their concentration lapses or they are distracted, they are likely to fall. Movement and activities are not smooth and natural in appearance. As children grow into adults, the pull of the spastic muscles may continue to be unbalanced which leads to increasing deformity of joints, so that although cerebral palsy is not progressive, it may look more severe or cause new or different problems.

Due to poor co-ordination of muscles, difficulties with breathing, speech and eating and drinking can occur. Most children with speech difficulties learn some kind of verbal communication while augmentative communication aids can help those with a more severe disability.

Certain difficulties and medical conditions are more common among people with cerebral palsy. They may also have to contend with epilepsy, vision, hearing or intellectual disabilities, bowel and bladder disorders and behavioural problems. Children with cerebral palsy may also have difficulties with learning, language, attention and memory.

Can cerebral palsy be treated?

Cerebral palsy is not a disease. It is not hereditary and it can occur in any family. Cerebral palsy cannot be cured but it is not a progressive condition. While it is not possible to repair the brain damage, much can be done throughout the life of a person to reduce the effect of cerebral palsy and improve their quality of life.*

*The information provided in 'What is cerebral palsy' is based on a booklet of the same name produced by The Spastic Centre of NSW.

Support services: Where to start

As Bradley points out, the carers of a person with disabilities often have a better understanding of the needs of that person than any one else. For that reason many also become expert at tracking down support services and facilities to suit their specific needs, but it is not always an easy task. Sometimes it requires a lot of detective work but the effort is well worth it if you find an organisation or individual who can provide the service you need, whether it be access to communication aids, advice on educational and employment opportunities, respite care — or simply someone to talk to.

For Sherron, by far the most valuable source of information is other parents. Sherron has learned not to be limited in exploring all possible options. She strongly believes that each parent or carer must have faith in themselves and their own responses to the needs of the child. They must continually question the 'experts' and seek empathetic professionals who are able to relate to the individual needs of each person. She believes that Unitems and Silence Isn't Golden have helped Bradley but is equally strong in her belief that each person must find his or her own truth.

Other useful sources of information and support include the local branch of the Department of Social Security, community health centres, local councils, regional centres for people with disabilities and general practitioners.

There are many organisations throughout Australia which offer support and services for people with cerebral palsy and their families. The Australian Cerebral Palsy Association operates a centre in each state capital. These are the first point of contact for a range of specialist facilities throughout the state. The contact details of each of these centres and a brief outline of some of their services are listed below. Several other related services, including those that Bradley and his family have found valuable, such as the Regency Park Centre for Young Disabled, MACAS (Microcomputer and Communication Aids Service) and the Make-a-Wish Foundation, are also listed.

The following is not designed to be an exhaustive directory, merely a starting point.

NEW SOUTH WALES & ACT

The Spastic Centre of New South Wales

PO Box 184

Brookvale NSW 2100

Ph: (02) 451 9022

The Spastic Centre of NSW offers a full range of services for babies, children and adults with cerebral palsy and their families in NSW and the ACT. The centre has compiled a comprehensive information directory called *Survival Guide for Parents* which lists services across the state and throughout Australia, ranging from resource centres, dial-a-mum support services, social work services, technical aids and toy libraries to holiday and travel options. It also runs an Assistive Device Service which provides information and advice on adaptive technology for people with disabilities and access to computers for vocational needs, education and leisure.

Computer Assessment Service

The NSW Society for Children and Young Adults

with Physical Disabilities

PO Box 4055

Parramatta NSW 2124

Ph: (02) 890 0100

The Computer Assessment Service is a resource centre which provides information and recommendations on micro-computer-based technology to people of all ages and with any disability. 'Technology' ranges from a simple on/off switch to sophisticated voice output communication devices and personal computer adaptations.

Technical Aid to the Disabled (TAD)

227 Morrison Road

Ryde NSW 2112

Ph: (02) 808 2022

TAD is a voluntary organisation dedicated to designing and making aids for adults and children with disabilities when such aids are not available commercially. Volunteers are skilled in areas such as design, engineering, medical and paramedical fields. TAD members do not charge for their services, but clients are asked, where possible, to cover the cost of materials. The organisation offers its services Australia wide.

Barrier Free Travel

36 Wheatley Street

North Bellingen NSW 2454

Ph: (066) 55 1733

Barrier Free Travel provides travel access information for people with disabilities, particularly those with mobility difficulties, who are planning to travel both within Australia and around the world. It is not a travel agent, but it provides information on accessible accommodation, transport and medical facilities.

NORTHERN TERRITORY

Carpentaria Community Services

GPO Box 4150

Darwin NT 0811

Ph: (089) 81 4040

Carpentaria Community Services (formerly the Northern Territory Spastics Association) offer a range of services to children and adults with cerebral palsy and other disabilities, and their families. Its programs include accommodation support, community access, early intervention, respite and attendant care, and personal and family support services.

QUEENSLAND

Queensland Spastic Welfare League

PO Box 386

Fortitude Valley QLD 4006

Ph: (07) 358 8011

Labrador Units: (075) 32 2088

The league provides a range of services to children and adults with cerebral palsy and other disabilities, including information, family support, early intervention, accommodation and employment support for adults, day programs, and specialised equipment and technology. It also provides holiday units at Labrador on the Gold Coast. These units are designed to cater for the specific needs of disabled people. Preference is given to clients of the league, but the units are available to interstate families.

MACAS (Microcomputer and Communication Aids Service)

PO Box 479

Stones Corner QLD 4120

Ph: (07) 394 7471

MACAS, a unit of the Independent Living Centre of Queensland, offers an unbiased information and advice service for people with disabilities regarding the use of technology, both equipment which has been developed for aiding those with specific disabilities and mainstream computers. It is unbiased because it has no links or commercial arrangements with manufacturers and therefore no obligation to recommend a specific brand or, indeed, to recommend the use of computer technology if it does not meet the individual's needs.

TASMANIA

Tasmanian Spastics Association

112 Gormanston Road

Moonah TAS 7009

Ph: (002) 72 0222

The Tasmanian Spastics Association offers services such as advice on employment opportunities, funding for medical services, transport, access to computers, technical aids and equipment and leisure activities.

Assistive Devices Clinic

Rehabilitation Tasmania

31 Tower Road

New Town TAS 7008

Ph: (002) 38 1812

The Assistive Devices Clinic specialises in augmentative communication devices for people with disabilities. Its services include adapting software, keyboards and other technology to suit specific needs, providing access to computer equipment and acting as a resource centre by keeping up to date on developments in other states and overseas in communications technology. The clinic also provides physiotherapy, occupational and speech therapy services.

SOUTH AUSTRALIA

Spastic Centres of South Australia Inc.

PO Box 49

Woodville SA 5011

Ph: (08) 268 5000

Spastic Centres of South Australia administer services in the city and country through regional offices. They offer a wide range of community-based services for people with disabilities, including accommodation, respite services, community access services and a disability awareness program which operates in schools, TAFE colleges, universities and service organisations.

The Crippled Children's Association of South Australia

Days Road

Regency Park SA 5010

Ph: (08) 243 8243

Regency Park Centre provides rehabilitation services for children and young people with a variety of severe physical disabilities, including cerebral palsy, spina bifida, neuromuscular disorders and traumatic injuries. Its facilities also include a Technology Assessment Service which offers advice and information on the use of computer technology to aid communication and for use in vocation, education and leisure activities.

VICTORIA

The Spastic Society of Victoria Ltd

135 Inkerman St

PO Box 381

St Kilda VIC 3182

Ph: (03) 537 2611

The Spastic Society of Victoria offers a range of services for children and adults, including employment and training services, residential services and leisure activities. The society produces various information booklets such as *Cerebral Palsy: A Brief Guide to the Facts and Myths* and *Parents are Therapists Too: A Parent's Guide.*

Microcomputer Application Centre (MAC)

Yooralla Society of Victoria

PO Box 88

South Melbourne VIC 3205

Ph: (03) 25 4566

A unit of the Yooralla Society of Victoria, the Microcomputer Application Centre (MAC) offers expert advice and information on communication technology for people with disabilities. This includes equipment which is designed to meet specific needs as well as mainstream computers.

Make-a-Wish Foundation

Registered Head Office

Suite 2, 315 Whitehorse Road

Balwyn VIC 3103

Ph: (03) 888 5762

    (008) 03 2260

The basic philosophy of the Make-a-Wish Foundation is to grant a child (under 18 years of age) with a life-threatening illness a special wish. Its aim is provide precious memories not only for the child, but their family and loved ones. Make-a-Wish has branches throughout Australia but the Victorian head office is the only one which operates full-time.

WESTERN AUSTRALIA

Cerebral Palsy Association of Western Australia Ltd

PO Box 61

Mt Lawley WA 6050

Ph: (09) 443 0211

The Cerebral Palsy Association of Western Australia offers a range of services for both children and adults with cerebral palsy. It offers therapy programs to help children develop the skills they require to participate in family, school and community life. Services for adults focus on helping them to participate in further education, employment and social activities. Where possible, programs are integrated into the community.

MACAS (Microcomputer and Communication Aids Service)

Independent Living Centre

3 Lemnos St

Shenton Park WA 6008

(09) 382 2011

Magic Is Within

We come into this world with nothing

and go out with exactly the same

And if we falter along the way we only

have ourselves to blame

At one time we've all let tears wipe

away the sadness from our face

And said or done things that make the

world a better place

We've all had special friends who give

a helping hand

The ones who truly love us and always

understand

We all need a purpose, an ambition or

direction to life-long goals

But we must remember that our bodies

are only casings for our souls

Sometimes things might get us down but

they only last a while

And nothing is ever too bad to take

away our smile

No matter what some say or do they

will never make us cry

For all we ever have to do in this

World is lie down and darn well die.

It doesn't matter if we're a pauper or

a movie star

It's what we've done with our lives

that determines who we are

And I'll blowed if I'll let them

write upon my epitaph:

'Here lies a loser who didn't have the

ability to laugh'.

Anyone can do anything they set their

mind to do

So let's start hearing about how your

dreams come true

There are three million other Bradley

stories somewhere out there

And a lot of other special people who

take the time to care.

Keep Smiling,

Bradley Harris Wolf